WHAT OTHERS ARE SAYING
ABOUT THIS BOOK:

"Jean is a person who dared to dream. You'll want to adopt her positive attitude after reading this book. Don't miss it."

-Richard Simmons
America's #1 Fitness Guru

"If you want to lose weight fast, read this book fast, and you will become who you want to be fast."

-Mark Victor Hansen
Co-creator of the #1 *New York Times* best-selling series: ***Chicken Soup for the Soul***

"Laughter is a wholesome, healthy thing. One hundred belly laughs a day and other sensible tips found in this book will bring longevity and humor to your life. I highly recommend it."

-Art Linkletter
TV Celebrity, Author of:
Kids Say the Darndest Things

"Before you can manage others, you must learn to manage yourself. This book will help you turn on, reward and energize yourself. You will experience increasing effectiveness. Make a commitment to read it!"

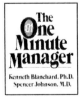

-Ken Blanchard
Co-author of #1 *New York Times* bestseller:
The One Minute Manager

"Take excellent care of your physical health. Jean's book will tell you how."

-Brian Tracy
Speaker, Author of 51 books, including:
The Psychology of Selling and *Maximum Achievement*

"Jean is a gifted communicator and has a passion for helping others to overcome their personal difficulties, as she has done herself."

-Florence Littauer
Founder of **CLASS**: Christian Leaders, Authors and Speakers Services. Author of 30 books including:
Personality Plus and *Silver Boxes*

"This book will stimulate, motivate and activate your ability to become the person you want to be. Jean's practical and encouraging words will make the difference for you. Read and enjoy, you'll never be the same again."

-Kathy Collard Miller
Speaker, Author of 42 books, including:
Why Do I Put So Much Pressure on Myself and *An Expressive Heart*

"I admire you so much for having walked through the darkness of the loss of loved ones, a serious illness and risen to your own magnificence. Your work is a ministry and your example has changed countless lives for the better. May your book deeply touch and inspire others to become all that our Divine Creator has seen for us."

-Reverend Peggy Price
Huntington Beach Church of Religious Science

"The message of this book is simple, effective and powerful. It is life-changing, as promised."
-Naomi Voorhees, Speaker, Author: *Head-On*

ABOUT THE AUTHOR

Have you ever wanted to reinvent yourself? Change your body? Your self-esteem? Your whole life?

If you're ready to make some changes—to live the life you truly want—to be all you <u>can</u> be—you must discover Jean Krueger's amazing success secrets.

Jean was living a nightmare. She was seriously overweight, in poor health and too exhausted and depressed to get out of bed. Then she made the decision to change. By combining her body, mind and spirit, she envisioned outrageous results. As the pounds dropped, her medical problems vanished. Her energy and enthusiasm skyrocketed. Jean's awesome 60-pound weight-loss success story was featured in **Reinventing Yourself With The Duchess of York**, a bestseller by Sarah Ferguson, The Duchess of York.

Now, Jean motivates others to change their lives, as well. Through her seminars and workshops, she inspires groups, churches and companies to lead healthy, happy and prosperous lives. A former college teacher, play director, and television producer, she won numerous awards. However, the work she does now is the most rewarding of all. *"It's like giving back life, itself,"* she says.

Jean was prompted to write this book because of her passion to tell others—what she did—they can do, too. This book reveals Jean's empowering strategies. Whatever it is you want to accomplish, you will learn how to tell yourself, *"I can do it!"* and then do it.

Dearest Nik,
Thank you soooo much for all your
support + creative ideas — I want to thank you

WHY THE WEIGHT?

for the gift that you are!

Dare To Be Great!

Jean Krueger

Light Works Publishing
Huntington Beach, California

Publisher's Cataloging-in-Publication
(Provided by Quality Books, Inc.)

Krueger, Jean.
    Why the weight? : dare to be great! / Jean Krueger.
    --1 st ed.
    p. cm.
    Includes bibliographical references and index.
    LCCN 2002094329
    ISBN 0-9722086-0-7

    1. Weight loss--Psychological aspects. 2. Obesity--
Psychological aspects. 3. Self-perception. 4. Mind and
Body. I. Title

RM222.2K78 2002   613.2'5'019
                         QB102-200651

Published by:
Light Works Publishing, 211 18 Street,
Huntington Beach, California 92648 U.S.A, 714-536-0408
skinnyjean@mindspring.com, or visit: www.allcalifspeakers.com

Cover Design by Herb Grondorf

Printed in the United States of America

CONTENTS

Acknowledgements
Foreword by Margaret Fishback Powers, Author of:
*Footprints, the Story Behind
the Poem That Inspired Millions*
Introduction by Becky Killian, Registered Dietitian

ACKNOWLEDGEMENTS

I extend my deepest gratitude to the following who helped to make this book possible: My husband, Dave, whose love, positive energy and support bolstered my body, mind and spirit; my daughter, Becky, from whom I continue to learn; my son, Kenny, whose energy is contagious; my grandchild, Nicole, whose enthusiasm kept me young; my sister, Mary, whose friendship I treasure; my sister-in-law, Mary, whose cheering was priceless; my sister-in-law, Diane, whose interest kept me going; my mother-in-law, Irene, and my brothers-in-law, Don, Ken and Tom, whose humor lifted me.

I feel fortunate and grateful for the many close friends who blessed me with their love, counsel, support and editing: Sally Beelner; Fran Berman; Karen Carrolls; Linda Chapman; Terry Cornelsen; Jane Crane; Kathleen Collard-Miller; Dolores Curry; Sandy Fazio; Eleanor S. Field, Ph.D.; Laara Gad; Barbara Hatton; Nedra Heller; Sharon Hood; Nik Jones; Nancy Kaehler; Katree; Darlene Kean; Linda Klein; Joanne LaChance; Suzanne Libertto; Martha Lockwood; Darlene March; Maria MacDonald; Joy Martin; Kay Nelson; Yvonne McGee; Vivian McKinley; Nancy Miller-Rounds; Mike Rounds; Lisa Mundy; Reverend Peggy Price; Carol Runzel; Stephen A. Scalf; Caroline Sean; Jane Shawber; Steve Smith, RScP; Lynn Stanford; Mark and Kathy Stern; Pauline Tedford, RScP; Christy Teague; Linda Thompson; Carlos Villanueva; Naomi Voorhees; Dottie Walters; Heather Wieshlow; Kathleen Yoder, and Sue Wilmot.

Heartfelt thanks go to Herb Grondorf for the cover design.

I would also like to express my deep appreciation to my friends and colleagues in Toastmasters, National Speakers Association, Mastermind, Friday Shirtsleeves, Creative Memories, Huntington Beach Church of Religious Science, my bridge groups, and my weight support groups members and staff. Without their friendship and support this book would still be only a dream.

FOREWORD

Dear Jean,

It is so difficult to overcome obstacles, isn't it, when you don't believe in yourself. You always expect the worst from yourself—and others, too! Then too, you can never really focus on a bigger goal, because you'll consistently be anxious about how you look, how others perceive you or whether you're going to <u>fail or fall</u>.

There's a power at work within each of us right now that can help us accomplish more that we could even ask or imagine. If we are just letting that power lay dormant because we don't recognize it, what then? Many are afraid to even claim it. How destructive low self-esteem can be to blind us to the power and the gifts that have been placed within us. Transfer that knowledge to others who have withdrawn and appear to have no hope.

There is a dream of trust that has become a path of faith with footprints to be followed that others may see and have confidence on their journey of hope. Someone has gone that way before and is sure and steady.

Now with hope of dreams realized and enthusiasm fulfilled, I pray you do great things as you follow in His footprints.

Following His Footprints daily,

Margaret Fishback Powers
Author of **FOOTPRINTS, The Story Behind
The Poem that Inspired Millions**

FOOTPRINTS—I Had a Dream

One night I dreamed a dream.
I was walking along the beach with my Lord.
Across the dark sky flashed scenes from my life
For each scene I noticed two sets
Of footprints in the sand,
One belonging to me, and one to my Lord.

When the last scene of my Life shot before me,
I looked back at the footprints in the sand.
There was only one set of footprints.
I realized that this was at the lowest
And saddest times of my life.
This always bothered me
And I questioned the Lord
About my dilemma.
"Lord, you told me when I decided to follow you,
You would walk and talk with me all the way.
But I was aware that during the most troublesome
Times of my life there is only one set of footprints.
I just don't understand why, when I needed you most
You leave me.
He whispered, "My precious child,
I love you and will never leave you.
Never, ever, during your trials & testings.
When you saw only one set of footprints
It was then that I carried you."

Margaret Fishback Powers

Used by special permission of the author, Margaret Fishback Powers, author of **FOOTPRINTS: The Story Behind the Poem That Inspired Millions**, and HarperCollins Publishers.

INTRODUCTION

Jean's book couldn't have come out at a better time. Obesity has reached epidemic proportions in the United States! The Surgeon General reports 62% of Americans are either overweight or obese. In 1980, that statistic was only 48%. (Obesity is often described as 30 pounds or more overweight.)

Overweight people experience a great deal more disease, and 44% higher health-care costs than people of normal weight. Carrying too much weight greatly increases your danger of developing many chronic conditions. Among these threats are high blood pressure, diabetes, heart disease, stroke, gall bladder disease, and cancer of the breast, prostate or colon. Obesity can lead to premature death. Each year, over 300,000 deaths in the U. S. are due to weight-related causes. Obesity is the second leading cause of preventable death. (Smoking is number one.)

As a nation, we have become more and more sedentary. We have also become extremely dependent upon fast foods and junk foods. What the American public doesn't know is these foods contain dangerous chemicals along with lots of fats, sugars and high calories. Not only do they add extra pounds, but they also deprive you of proper nutrition. They clog your body and deprive your mind (and spirit) of the energy and nutrients necessary to achieve your life's goals. Therefore, your weight can be the one thing that gets in the way of everything.

The fresh fruits, vegetables and other healthy foods mentioned in this book help your body to function at its optimum level. Most of them contain fiber, which will keep you satisfied so you won't crave the junk foods. By eating the foods suggested in this book, you will find your ideal weight. The antioxidants and vitamins these foods contain will also help prevent aging, heart disease, cancer, high blood pressure, high cholesterol and a host of other problems.

Since the disaster of 9/11/01, our nation's collective waistband has widened. With our tragic loss of humanity, many have abandoned their diets and are eating their emotions, instead. Many experienced a tragic loss of their loved ones. Unfortunately, emotional eating can result from a feeling of loss of any type, including: loss of self-esteem, loss of a job, loss of feeling needed, and loss of goals. Happily, Jean's book also deals with steps to giving closure to any loss that may have led to emotional eating, and to finding the positives in everything. This book is a blueprint to leading a happier, healthier and more active life.

The sensible tips found in this book will lead to fitness of your body, mind and spirit. I highly recommend you read it. ***WHY THE WEIGHT? Dare To Be Great!***

~Becky Killian, *Registered Dietitian*~

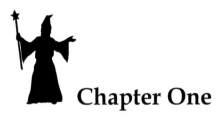

Chapter One

The Magic In You

Are you overweight? Does your excess weight stop you from achieving your ultimate self-image and success? Do you struggle with the scale, yet you don't even know why you're overweight? Do you find yourself spending money on clothing in sizes you don't even want to be wearing? Are you missing out on job opportunities? Life opportunities?

This book changes your life and rescues your dreams. You are about to produce something magical—a new you! Get ready to transform your life on all levels—body mind and spirit. This book makes your life enriched. It makes your life easier to live. This book makes you a better person. Read it and your life will change! I promise. You have all the magical powers you need within you right now. Why the wait? ***WHY THE WEIGHT? DARE TO BE GREAT!***

The Surgeon General has proclaimed 62% of Americans are overweight or obese. Are you among them? Read and learn secrets to produce stunning weight-loss results in the next twenty-one days. In this book you discover:

- How to eat more, yet weigh less. (See Chapter 5.)
- How to lose five pounds instantly with a magical soup. (See page 150.)

- Fifty-One Fat-Burning Foods that will shape you to your ideal weight. (Don't miss Chapter 6.)
- On the spot "**SUCCESS** *formula.*" (See page 86.)
- Seven Keys to a slimmer you. (Turn to Chapter 7.)
- Four Agreements that will change your world.
- One-Hundred-and-One Weight-Loss Secrets.
- PLUS, how to say: *"I can do it,"* and then DO it, and much, much MORE...

You have been waiting for this book! Get ready. You are about to discover the recipe for your weight-loss success.

I reshaped my entire life, and I will show you how to do the same. Read this book and learn how I lost sixty pounds by eating more! I changed my life and enjoyed every minute of it. My high blood pressure and cholesterol are gone. I look and feel twenty years younger. Best of all, I no longer go to food for comfort. I learned food should not be used to hide emotions, but rather to celebrate life. Now I enjoy food more than ever. What I have done, you can do, too. Read on, and discover the secrets.

After experiencing the losses of the most important people in my life, I knew what it was like to "eat" my emotions. My life had been a pattern of adversity, yet I pulled through. I proved to myself that I was an unsinkable soul.

This book is offered as encouragement to countless others who carry weight—not just on their hips, but also in their hearts and on their shoulders. I hope I can touch their lives by baring my soul. Using the same courage, I hope you will do the same. I know how easy it is to turn to food for the answer. I knew I had a book inside of me, with a message that could inspire others. At last, with the help of family and friends, here it is. So I ask you, **WHY THE WEIGHT? Dare To Be Great!** Right now!

The Connection

Think about it. Suppose your car has a spiffy new engine and a full tank of gas, but it doesn't have brakes. It isn't drivable, is it? Or imagine your car has a fast motor, and it can stop on a dime, but it doesn't have gas. It's still not drivable, right? If your car has good brakes and a full tank of gas, but your motor doesn't run, it still isn't drivable.

If one thing is lacking, nothing works. If your motor doesn't run, it doesn't matter how much gas your car has, or how reliable your brakes are...all three have to be functioning. They are all interconnected.

Body, mind and spirit are all connected, in the same way. If your spirit is lacking, your body and mind suffer, too. If your mind is muddled, your body and spirit lack clarity, also. If your body is burdened by extra weight, your mind and spirit follow suit. **YOUR WEIGHT CAN BE THE ONE THING THAT TOUCHES UPON EVERYTHING ELSE!** Extra pounds can stop you from achieving all your other dreams.

Many things can get in the way of your body, mind and spirit working together. For instance, you may have suffered a loss. Consider your emotions and how you handled them if you have experienced any of the following:

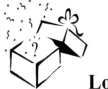

Loss = Gain

- Loss of health
- Loss of respect for a person you admired or loved
- Loss of your own self-esteem, stemming from an abusive relationship

- Loss of physical ability
- Loss of familiar friends and places as a result of a move
- Loss of something stolen or misplaced
- Loss of a family pet
- Loss of finances
- Loss of youth
- Loss of a job
- Loss of self-esteem
- Loss of goals and importance stemming from retirement
- Loss of feeling needed due to "empty-nest" syndrome
- Loss of self
- Loss of faith in God
- Loss of faith in yourself
- Loss of faith in others
- Loss or separation of a relationship
- Loss of a loved one through death
- Loss of security
- Loss of humanity

Each of the above losses may be experienced to the same depth felt in grieving a loss or death of a loved one. Losses cause you to seek comfort. Experiencing grief from a loss can cause you to go to the **COMFORT OF FOOD**, thinking it will soothe you.

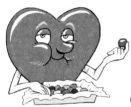

Comfort is Not Happiness

Food anesthetizes you. Food calms and quiets your emotions within. Food can become your drug of choice. Regrettably, when you suffer the death of a loved one, food arrives before the funeral even begins. Unfortunately, food can become an enormous sabotage, and can create a weight gain. But it never heals or fills the emptiness in your heart.

I know. For a long time, I felt tremendously angry with God. I blamed Him for all my problems and hurts, and especially for the losses I suffered as an adult twelve years ago, when my Mom, my Dad and my three brothers all died. Because their deaths were so close together, (three of them within eight months of each other), I never knew for whom I was mourning. Yet I felt like I was continually bleeding inside. Food became my comforter and my friend.

I was overwhelmed with grief. I tried to shut out my feelings and short-circuit my pain. I tried to keep busy so I wouldn't experience the loneliness, and heartache. All the while, I ate as if I could never fill myself up.

Eventually, I found myself crying unexpectedly at any time. Frightened, I felt something was terribly wrong with me. Finally, I joined two bereavement groups—one at my church and the other at a local hospital. I wish I had sought out this type of support immediately after the death of my Dad, who was the first to die. I learned people normally go through many of the same stages of emotions when they suffer a loss. I was not alone with these heavy feelings:

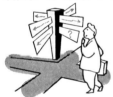

The "Weighty" Stages of Loss

- Shock and denial—"Oh, no, it can't be!"
    (I could close my eyes, picture their faces and hear their voices. They couldn't be dead! At first, I was totally numb.)
- Deep feelings of sadness, sorrow, emptiness and loss of meaning and purpose in life.
    (I felt as if I was continually bewildered, aching, and torn from inside.)
- A restless need for activity, yet finding it difficult to concentrate.
    (I went back to school, signed up for a full-time load, and resumed teaching at the same

time. I kept so busy I neglected my family and myself. I didn't want to face my feelings or be alone with them.)

- Aimless wandering, forgetfulness, unfinished tasks.
  (All my "busy-ness" was fretful and useless.)
- Difficulty with eating, either loss of appetite or overeating.
  (No problem with loss of appetite! Food became my drug of choice.)
- An uncontrollable need to cry often and at unexpected times.
  (I wore sunglasses at all times. I remember breaking into tears and sobbing in the canned goods aisle of the supermarket, when I merely picked up a can of peas. I never knew why or what hit me. I learned later, crying is a necessary biological process. It's good to keep crying until you can't.)
- Protecting others who seem uncomfortable around you by not talking about your feelings of loss, even when the need to talk is greatest.
  (This was my biggest problem. I stuffed down all my emotions of guilt, sorrow and loneliness with food. I needed desperately to share my feelings and get them out, instead. I wanted to tell others what I needed and didn't need from them, yet I couldn't muster the courage.)
- Guilt over things that happened or didn't happen, that were said or not said.
  (Guilt was definitely a major reaction for me. I kept telling myself: "I SHOULD HAVE called more often..." or "I SHOULD HAVE told them how much I loved them..." or "I SHOULD HAVE flown back home more often..." I "SHOULD HAVE" all over myself!)
- Anger at your loved one for leaving, or hostility toward others.
  (Anger is a way through the sadness. This is one stage of grief I never went through. I never felt the anger I was supposed to feel. Maybe I held it all inside. If I had allowed myself to feel rage or even resentment, I may not have

sabotaged and anesthetized myself with food as I did. I never actually finished the cycle of my grief. I found out later to abandon feelings is not the way to health. To cut short your grieving process is to shortcut the wisdom you can gain from experiencing a loss. Unfortunately for me, I chose to go around my grief, not through it.)

The bereavement counselor at my church warned me eventually I would feel rage. I never did. I only postponed, and prolonged my pain and hurt. Now I know with pain there is healing. I was not willing to experience the pain, so I only delayed the inevitable.

Then came even more loss...my own cancer and a painful removal of my kidney, followed by the loss of my all-time favorite job as a television producer/writer. Next, my husband lost his job as a CEO in a corporate-merger. During all these darkest moments of my soul, I sensed God had left me. I felt alone and forsaken. It wasn't anger; it was a feeling of numbness. Yet I truly needed to find peace within my heart, and to rediscover my inner spirit. Instead, I went to food.

Years later, I discovered the famous poem, ***Footprints--I Had a Dream*** by Margaret Fishback Powers. The verse described someone who also questioned why God left him during the lowest and saddest times in his life. The final line exploded in front of me, like a personal message:

> *"...He whispered, 'My precious child,*
> *I love you and will never leave you.*
> *Never, ever, during your trials and testings.*
> *When you saw only one set of footprints,*
> *it was then that I carried you.'"*

I suddenly realized I had the spiritual support I needed, all along. It was I who had turned away. Now, you may do that too, but it only prolongs the grieving process. If you are strong enough to stop old destructive judgments and not let them hinder you in anyway, you will help facilitate the healing.

Part of my self-destruction stemmed from my fear that people were judging me, especially about my brothers, Jerry and Jeff, who died from AIDS, and my other brother Jack, who died because of suicide. At the time, my mother didn't want to tell anyone what had happened, nor would she attend their funerals. She referred to the causes of my brothers' deaths as "cancer," and a "gunshot wound."

My brothers, Jerry and Jeff, who both died after a courageous battle with AIDS, left me with a terrible regret for a tragic interruption of their gifted young lives. They were so creative—so full of promise. After their deaths, I felt I had to fight the stigma people may have had in the back of their minds about their disease. I found myself being judged, yet I may have been my own worst judge.

"Weight" of What Others Think

Terry Cole Whittaker says it all in her book: *What You Think of Me is None of My Business.* She tells how too often, we use our perceptions of people's opinions of us to make ourselves feel guilty, wrong, or inadequate. Other people who say insensitive things or think disapproving beliefs about you is their own little drama in which YOU play only a MINOR part! Remember: what other people say about you, what other people think about you, is NONE OF YOUR BUSINESS—because it's about them, not you! Why worry about what other people think—most aren't even thinking about you, anyway. You have your own play in which to star. Love yourself, and know God doesn't make junk. I know now, I needed to fill myself with God, not food.

I was overcome with sorrow, yet I wondered if I was over-reacting in my grief. I chose to isolate and insulate myself. I refused to talk with and share with the people who could help me the most. Because my brothers' deaths had no real burials, I could not experience any real closure. Yet my fingers were not broken. I could have picked up a phone at anytime. A support group would have been an excellent place to share my feelings. Instead, I chose to busy myself, escape, and try to heal that way.

My brother, Jack, who took his own life, left an endless trail of questions that begged for answers. Somehow I felt I never truly knew him. I never discovered any satisfactory explanations. Yet I discovered the plight of all suicide survivors in a struggle to break free of its stigma.

I felt guilty about everything related to his loss. All those times I misread and was hurt by his seeming disinterest in me or what I had to say, I could have been more compassionate and knowing. He was the one who was depressed and in deep pain. Instead, I allowed myself to feel hurt. How foolish!

Why didn't I hear the hopelessness in his voice, and know he was about to make his last choice? I am still puzzled, perplexed and wondering what he was thinking. I try to see things from his point of view. I could focus on all the tragic memories, except now, in retrospect, I would rather recall the happier moments we knew together as kids.

You can think of a million reasons to feel guilty when a person takes his own life. I was too blinded by what *I thought* was happening. I was hesitant to interfere. I could have called more often. I could have had my kids call him more often. I could have urged my husband to call him.

God forgives those things of which we are guilty. If He forgives, we should too. At the time, I needed to allow myself more compassion. Instead, I ate more hamburgers. Sometimes described as the "ultimate personal rejection" (no wonder Mom and I resorted to food) suicide thrusts survivors into a jumble of emotional confusion, different from nearly every other kind of bereavement. The main problem is—there are no definite warning signs. There is always twenty-twenty hindsight, but suicide is never altogether predictable by anyone until it has happened.

That's when both Mom and I really missed dad, who had died a few years earlier. Dad was my hero and cheerleader on the field of life. I thought dad would be forever. When he died of prostate cancer, the impact of his death was overwhelming. Because his cancer went into remission several times, I felt like we lost him over and over.

Now, living in different states, Mom and I both stuffed down our emotions with food, and tried to fill something you could never fill—a hole in your heart. Within a few months after my brothers' deaths, she died too. The doctor said my mother died of a blood clot. Deep down, I believe she died because of weight-related causes from a broken heart. I grieved once again the sorrow of her death and all the guilt that went along with having an aging parent, out-of-town and out-of-touch.

Since then I learned to have more compassion for myself, and to be open to the healing process. I needed to "break down" before I could "break through." I accepted life will never be the same as before, and I forgave myself, realizing I was not responsible for all that had happened. I learned I was only responsible for how I choose to deal with what happened. Life goes on. I found I could expand my circle of activities and acquaintances, and actually add years to my own life. I learned out of every loss comes a gain. (Rather than a weight gain, you can experience a life gain, if you are open to it.) I finally realized I could begin a new life, and experience renewed body, mind and spirit because I found:

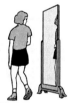

The New Me

I always dreamed of being slim, like I used to be in high school. That was just a dream, however. The reality, on the other hand, was ever since those high school days, I started living a tremendously unhealthy lifestyle.

I struggled with my weight ever since my college days filled with bratwurst, beer and fast food. Now, I was in my fifties, with two grown children, and a grandchild. I was hit with arthritis, heel spurs, asthma and high blood pressure. My doctor warned me my cholesterol was climbing. I had been taking high blood-pressure medication for years.

When I surpassed my husband's weight, I knew it was time to do something. Instead, I went into denial. I just stopped weighing myself, and bought bigger and bigger muumuus. Most mornings, I used to wait to get out of bed until my husband left the room. I didn't want him to see me struggle to get up, to get dressed, or to bend over.

Finally I experienced a "wake-up" moment. In January of 1998, I saw a picture someone took of me that I thought was my mother. (Photos of me were quite rare, because I was usually the photographer. I would always hide from anyone else taking pictures.) I thought my weight gain was my little secret. Finally, I realized the whole world knew too.

I stared and glared at that photo. I looked so old. I looked as old as my mother did when she died, and that was almost ten years earlier. The incident scared me. I decided I wanted far more in my life than to die early, like she did. The year 1998 was going to be the year of the "NEW ME." I was determined to change on every level—body, mind and spirit.

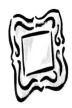

Shaping Dreams

Once this realization set in, I spent a day in seclusion, listening to inspirational tapes. Next, I asked myself some hard questions:

- WHO would I like to become?
  I always wanted to be someone who made a difference in people's lives.
- WHERE would I like to go?
  I dreamed of going to Hawaii, the Caribbean and to cruise to exotic places.
- WHAT would I like to create in my life?
  I wanted to generate good feelings, like happiness and laughter.
- WHAT would I like to do in my life?
  I wanted to use my creative talents of speaking and writing to my highest vision.

- WHAT skills and abilities did I want to master?
  I thought of things I had never done: scuba diving, bike riding, and stock investing.
- WHAT character traits did I want to develop?
  I longed to be confident, easy-going, interesting, friendly, likeable and loveable.
- WHAT career goals did I have for myself?
  I dreamed of becoming a famous speaker and writer.
- WHAT did I need to do to feel good about myself physically?
  I wanted to lose weight, and to gain energy and confidence through exercise.
- WHAT did I need to do to feel good about myself intellectually?
  I needed to read more books, newspapers and be open to more things.
- WHAT did I need to do to feel good about myself spiritually?
  I needed to find, talk to, listen to and serve God. Also to see Him in others.
- WHAT did I need to do to feel good about myself financially?
  I needed to produce a real income, learn to invest wisely, and to worry less.
- WHAT did I need to do to feel good about myself socially?
  I wanted to feel I belonged and was accepted. I wanted positive friends in my life.
- WHAT did I need to do to feel good about myself personally?
  I longed for self-esteem, peace, patience, and a better reflection in the mirror.
- WHAT did I need to do to feel good about myself professionally?
  I needed not to be afraid of marketing my talents, my abilities and myself.
- WHAT would I like to do or be in one year? Five years? Twenty?

I didn't know how to answer those questions, because I could hardly imagine losing five pounds, let alone sixty. Yet,

I could see my weight was the **ONE** thing that interfered with **EVERYTHING**! Nonetheless, I sat and wrote and wrote. I drew up goals that ignited my passions. I set dates and objectives on every level. It was going to be a new life.

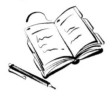

The Action Plan

Next, I made a date with myself to join a weight support group. You see, I tried to lose weight alone before and failed miserably. It wasn't until I attended a support group regularly I found the accountability and inspiration I needed to keep me going. There are many groups from which to choose. You might try Richard Simmons (check out his website—it's fabulous!), Overeaters Anonymous, Weigh Down, Weight Watchers, TOPS (Take Off Pounds Sensibly), or form a group of like-minded people, yourself.

When I came home from my first meeting (I'm referring to this time around, not the other three times when I became a dropout) I decided I was going to actually make it work. I was ready to do whatever I had to do to make it happen. (At this point, I would have eaten mud, if it were necessary— that's how committed I was.) This time I would truly take the time to read everything I could get my hands on about nutrition, weight-loss and exercising regularly. It was all worth the effort. This was something I had never done before. (I think the other three times I joined, I thought I would lose weight by just showing up, or by osmosis, or something.)

Over the course of that year, 1998, I worked relentlessly at peeling sixty pounds from my five-foot five-inch frame. I figured it took time to put the weight on; it would take time to take the weight off. A year would pass anyway, and it was worth it. I was worth it!

In order to accomplish that, I needed to change my environment. I decided to get all "red light" foods out of sight. Pizza had to go. It was one food I knew I could never stop at a single piece, because one piece meant three or four. I never had pizza again for a full year and a half. I also asked my husband to support me in my efforts and to hide his cashews and chips in his sock drawer, or the garage or someplace too high or low for me to reach.

I told him I would no longer be bringing home snacks that were a sabotage to me, and if he needed them, he could buy them himself, and to please hide them. (Incidentally, my husband, who had gained weight, as I had, through the thirty-some years of our marriage, lost twenty pounds, just by being in the new environment of our kitchen.)

I decided this time I was going to take the time to plan, time to shop, and time to read labels. I was shocked to find some of my old favorites, things I thought were wise and healthy choices (like chili relleno), had thirty-two grams of fat! Even Caesar and Chef Salads packed a big "fat" punch. I soon challenged myself to find things with higher fiber counts, lower fat and lower calorie counts.

Another thing I wanted to do was to become more open-minded and try new things like red beets, salads, beans and fruits. These were things I never liked as a child. Each week I decided to try a new fruit or vegetable. Soon I found I was doing most of my shopping at farmer's markets for lots of fruits and veggie. I also shopped health food stores for non-fat soy milk, and soy burgers (things I found were good for me as a cancer survivor) and low-fat tofu (good for hot flashes and a potential natural hormone replacement.) One of my favorite breakfasts was a smoothie made in the blender with fruits, non-fat soymilk and tofu. The energy it provided would often hold me until noon.

For lunch, I often put together my favorite sandwich: bean sprouts, cucumbers, tomatoes, spinach, avocado, mustard and a sprinkle of garlic powder on a dense wheat bread. This satisfied me, and I found I had plenty of calories left for later. If I was still hungry, I loaded up on more veggies.

At supper, I ate three to four ounces of chicken, or six to eight ounces of fish. I started to think of proteins more as a condiment than as a main entrée. The veggies with potato, whole grained bread or pasta became the main event. (I found too much protein could possibly take calcium from other nutrients or from your bones, in order for your body to digest it.) Beef and pork were things I avoided because of their higher fat content. Soon I felt the difference. I was feeling less tired and sluggish.

Nighttime snacks were popcorn or diet puddings along with high fiber cereal with cherries or other fruit. With the crunch, the sweetness and the fullness they'd provide, I felt like I was having "Rocky Road" ice cream.

The best lesson I learned was I could still be a volume eater! (I am to this day, but now I fill up on the right things.) I learned this secret at my first meeting from a woman who won an award for losing fifty pounds. She turned to the rest of us and said, "I eat a potato each day the size of my shoe!" That was the greatest news I ever heard. Potatoes were the kind of comfort food I craved. I filled up on them along with salsa, mushrooms, broccoli, sprouts, and spray butter. I made a whole meal of it.

Let me share a secret with you—spray butter. I just can't say enough about it. It certainly saved me. Being a girl from Wisconsin, I developed horrible habits of slathering on butter, sour cream, gravy, sauces and cheese. Now I use spray butter instead, on everything: vegetables, fish, toast, and popcorn. I take it everywhere—to friends' homes, to restaurants, even to the movies. (When I go to the movies, I bring my own popcorn, too. No one ever stops me. Of course, I don't flaunt it, yet if they ever ask me, I'm ready with an answer: I'm allergic to their movie popcorn—it makes me break out all over—in FAT!)

I found myself more assertive when I ate out in restaurants. I was surprised to find waiters were happy to accommodate most requests. I asked that my fish be broiled or grilled with little or no oil; my eggs be egg whites, prepared light, and "skip the cheese please." (All I needed was the moisture from the cheese, and I'd bring my spray butter for that. "No butter on the bread or toast, and put my salad dressing or sauce on the side?")

Previously, I ordered extra tartar sauce and salad dressings before I even started my meal. Now I had plenty left when I finished. This change was due thanks to the "fork trick," something I also learned from a fellow support-group member. With my dressing "on the side" I could use a fork to pick up only the flavor on the tines of the fork, and then I speared the food. A small amount of dressing provided all I needed of a wonderful, satisfying taste.

Mexican restaurants were always my favorite. Now they presented a special challenge because even if I made a good choice from the menu, I sabotaged myself with all the chips that came before my entrée arrived. So, I started asking the waiter to bring sliced cucumbers for me to dip along with the chips and salsa he brought for everyone else.

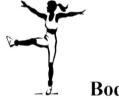

Body Fitness

My new exercise habits were also a big part of my weight loss. I had little interest in exercise before. I always figured it was a waste of time. *(I had more important things to do with my time, right? Ha!)* Now I see, when I look at my old picture—THAT was the waste of time! Since my support-group leader emphasized exercise, I figured I'd start with something easy. I was in a lot of pain with arthritis in my hip and heel spurs in my feet. I signed up for aqua-aerobics one day a week. Since we lived a block from the beach, I also started walking barefoot at low tide, or biking the beach trails for a few miles on the other days.

What a difference exercise made. I felt great! I saw results immediately—not only in how energized I felt, but also in my weight-loss progress. I soon increased to three days of aqua-aerobics, and started taking longer and longer walks and bike rides. I found exercise was fun. It was easy and didn't have to cost a lot of money. Whatever cost I incurred, I said, "I'm worth it!" I was also worth the time invested because I loved what exercise did for me. I found later, that investing an hour a day to some type of exercise is the best investment of time I can make toward a happier, healthier, longer life. (After all, if we eat every day, we want to exercise every day, too.)

When I lost twenty-five pounds, I decided I wanted to go to San Diego and join the twenty-mile "Midnight Madness Fun Ride" along the streets and beaches of that beautiful city. It was a way to see a scenic route not open to bikers at any other time, and to experience a new adventure with other bikers. They were competing for prizes—not for speed—but for creativity. Sporting pajamas and teddy bears, they lit up not only themselves, but also their bikes. My husband and I joined them and felt younger than we had in years.

The next adventure was the fifty-mile "Rosarita-Ensenada Fun Ride." I loved the word "fun-ride" because it was not a race—rather a great experience with light-hearted people who liked to exercise and liked to party. What a wonderful combination. Yet how challenging was the two-and-a-half mile stretch up a seven-and-a-half percent grade of El Tigre Mountain– the name described it all. Yet I was determined to complete the entire ride by pedaling every step of the way. I have to admit I was amazed at my own endurance and persistence when people far younger, and more able-bodied than I was, either walked their bikes or gave up. Many took the "sag" wagon, a truck, which followed the route to pick up those who faded and wanted out.

I remember, one beautiful young girl, clad in a scant bikini, whom I passed several times as she walked her bike on some of the roughest hills. Her comment to me, as I pedaled by at sometimes only 3 miles per hour was, "You go, girl!" Wow! Her words just made my heart sing.

When I lost thirty-five pounds, my leader's challenge to us was to try things we had always dreamed of doing, yet never got to do. I always wanted to scuba dive. I told my husband,

and the next thing I knew, we were signed up to become certified divers! Carrying a twenty-four pound weight-belt around my waist and fifty-pound air tank on my back were feats I could never have accomplished earlier that year with all the weight I carried. Now, my biggest obstacle was to get rid of my fear of drowning.

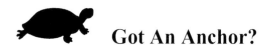 ## Got An Anchor?

That was where my anchor came in handy. (An anchor is a mental strategy. You use an image or object to recall a strong feeling.) I chose the calmness of the turtle, an animal I admired for its slow-moving grace, to think of during my weight-loss journey. When I approached a buffet table loaded with goodies, the composure of the turtle got me through many temptations, slowed my actions and helped me keep control. I gained new awe and respect of the turtle from a dive master who told me he copied the peace of mind of the turtle in his training on free dives over ninety-feet deep. He told me the turtle is one animal that uses less oxygen than any other, because it conserves its energy.

So, once again, I used the same anchor I used for my weight loss, but this time for my diving—the peacefulness of the turtle. That serenity helped me overcome my fear of the water and the waves and to gather my courage to trust myself. With that, I plunged beneath the surface to find what wonders awaited me there. It took me several failures and aborted dives before I got certified, but it was well worth it!

My husband and I have gone on the trips of our dreams, since then, to wonderful places like the Grand Cayman, the Caribbean and Catalina, to experience awesome fish and coral, stingrays and eels. It's like we're in a science fiction film, and we are the stars.

After I reached my goal-weight, I used my anchor once again, which incidentally, saved my life. My husband and I were diving off Catalina Island. When we surfaced, we found we were in heavy afternoon whitecaps. We were both swept into the rocks by a heavy surge. My husband broke his hand, (something he didn't know at the time). I broke my arm and dislocated my shoulder. I couldn't move my arm, which was stuck in a rock, and I sensed something was dreadfully misaligned. Another wave came and knocked my air supply out of my mouth, and yet another wave knocked my mask off my face. I couldn't see. I choked down water, trying to breathe. I tried to move my arm to find my air tube and my mask, but my broken arm was immobile. Sputtering, I was almost out of breath, as more and more waves crashed over my head.

All my fears of drowning returned. I wanted desperately to thrash about to help myself. It was then, I told myself to breathe slowly and be relaxed like the turtle. With my eyes shut, I stopped my frenzy and slowly felt for my air supply and found it with my good arm. Still unable to see, I coolly continued to feel for my mask, while clinging onto the rocks. Soon, I felt arms reaching me, removing my fins, air tank and weight belt. They were lifting me to higher ground.

My husband had pulled himself to the rocks above to shed his heavy gear, so he could come back down and help me. We were taken by helicopter to Long Beach, where my arm and shoulder and Dave's hand were set twelve hours later. Between my fear of drowning and the pain of bone clanging against bone all those hours, I was grateful for the anchor of calmness I developed in breathing and moving like a turtle.

Milestones

Back to my weight-loss journey—I had some great milestones along the way. The first was I lost twelve pounds. Twelve pounds was significant to me because it meant I was serious. I had joined a weight-loss support group three times before. I would lose ten pounds, and then lose interest because the friend I joined with dropped out. So I always dropped out, too. That was my level of commitment before. Now, this time I didn't tell anyone I was joining because I was still afraid of failure. But this time was different because this time I wanted it for me. It wasn't until I lost twenty-five pounds that I told anyone. Then half my bridge club joined. I wished I had told them earlier, because I wouldn't have had to go the journey alone.

There's a life's lesson here—**DON"T HIDE YOUR DREAM.** Others become attracted to your vision and want to come along.

My next milestone occurred when I returned from a cruise. I had lost twenty pounds before we left. I was certainly excited—it was my first cruise. I was also scared I would gain the weight back. Yet when I returned, I found I actually lost weight. What a triumph! Of course, as I see it, I learned a new lifestyle by then. I was determined to exercise each day by taking the stairs, and showing up for every exercise class available aboard ship. I ordered from the light side of the menu, and of course, I took my spray butter along.

Then, other things happened. I bought a sexy black skirt, yet I could only wear it for ten minutes at a time. It was so tight—it hurt. It wasn't until a few months later I tried it on, and it almost fell to the floor. What a thrill! I didn't mind the money for that outfit went to waste. (Or is it waist?) I learned then to let go of an old mind-set about waste. For instance, money wasn't going to waste if I didn't buy the economy-size because I was trying to learn portions. I didn't need to buy what was on-sale, when it had too many calories or too much fat. I told myself: "going to waste in reality means going to 'waist'." After experiencing success, I reminded myself: "**NOTHING TASTES AS GOOD AS THIN FEELS!**"

The most wonderful feeling came the day I took a bunch of my old clothes to a consignment store. That action was symbolic to me. I was saying goodbye to a chapter to which I would never return. I used the money for clothes in a new trim size—things with belts, and a waist—stylish fitting things that fit snuggly and encouraged me to suck-in and tuck-in my tummy.

I also started to take on a new posture. I could tell the way I carried myself reflected my new attitude, and I felt great. If ever I caught myself slumped over, I straightened immediately. I felt a new sense of happiness, and unstoppable power come over me. I found it was impossible to feel bad on the inside if I showed happiness on the outside, and vice-versa.

Miraculously, after slimming down, all my health problems disappeared. My doctor said I no longer needed the high-blood-pressure pills. My asthma was gone, too. My heel spurs no longer bothered me. I was leading an incredibly active lifestyle. Losing weight became a catalyst for all kinds of other challenges I wanted to tackle in my life. I kept working to change on all levels—physically, intellectually, emotionally, socially and spiritually. I continued to motivate myself to strive to be the best person I could possibly be.

Intellectually I tried to be open to all things. I read more than I used to. I kept abreast of the stock market. I listened to motivational tapes all the time. I now had more friends in my life who were positive and supportive. I surrounded myself with encouraging people who would help me grow. I worked at becoming a better friend, a better wife and a better listener—by being me. I looked at the glass now, as being half full. I tried to see the best in people rather than things I might have been judging them for in the past.

I had no idea what the benefits of getting slim were. Waddling around with all that weight had imprisoned me in so many ways. My new health and energy level amazed me. I began to look twice when I saw my own reflection. I continually wondered—who is that woman wearing my dress?

I also found I could change myself on many other levels. I discovered there were more facets to me and more heights I could reach. I used to get caught up on a treadmill of life, not unlike a hamster running on a wheel. I didn't take time to enjoy life. It was always rush, rush, rush. I never stopped to think about my goals and how to realize them. Now I found I reacted to people and things so differently. I didn't have the bad feelings I used to have. I took time to think about being thankful. I started to keep a gratitude journal, and each night before I went to bed, I wrote down five things I was grateful for that happened that day.

Oh! What a Feeling!

All of a sudden, one day, I was told I reached my weight goal. Wow, what a feeling of personal triumph! The next thing I knew, my leader was asking me if I would like to join the staff. It was a question that came at an appropriate time because I had been semi-retired for a couple of years. I was in truth missing my old days of teaching, and I had thought over and over of going back to it. Teaching had been a way of helping others, something I had always enjoyed. I always felt through my teaching, I had a way of bringing out the very best in my students—to improve their writing, or public speaking, or acting, or whatever the subject matter. This would be a way of giving back life, itself. Now that I had found a new life, and twenty years of lost youth, I wanted to impart that gift to others, as well!

Next I was chosen as a weight-loss media-ambassador. I appeared on numerous television shows and was invited to speak to large audiences to share my tips for success. Then my success story was featured in the best-selling book, *Reinventing Yourself With The Duchess of York*, written by Sarah Ferguson, The Duchess of York. Indeed, I have reinvented myself. I am aspiring to change on all levels, and I'm not done yet. It's so exciting because I don't know what's going to happen next. All my big dreams are coming true.

I continue to listen to master motivators like Mark Victor Hansen, Jack Canfield, Ken Blanchard, and numerous others. They spark remarkable philosophies, techniques and sound values I use to propel me to the speaking and writing career and life of which I always dreamed. As a result, this book is filled with helpful strategies, secrets and common sense. Watch out. **IT WILL CHANGE YOUR LIFE!**

Metamorphosis

The past few years have turned my dreams into reality, one I treasure deeply. I've gone through a metamorphosis. The roly-poly caterpillar is gone and in its place is a butterfly. I've got a brand new life—a whole new me. When I look back, I don't think I actually liked myself when I was heavy. Now I like myself a lot, and I love my life. I think I used to use food as a substitute for truly living. Those food binges are over. Now, I'm bingeing on life.

That's why you dream differently, as you let go of any extra burden you carry. You are inspired to reach for your optimum potential. You continue to aspire higher and higher to fulfill your heart's desires. You find you are open to more new things to keep on improving your life. Just change ONE THING—your weight—and you change everything—body, mind and spirit. They are all connected.

Take time to ask yourself the same questions that changed my life. May they cause you to "Dare to Dream" and change your body, mind and spirit, as well:

- WHO would I like to become?
- WHERE would I like to go?
- WHAT would I like to create in my life?
- WHAT would I like to do in my life?
- WHAT skills and abilities do I want to master?
- WHAT character traits do I want to develop?
- WHAT career goals do I have for myself?
- WHAT do I need to do to feel good about myself physically?
- WHAT do I need to do to feel good about myself intellectually?
- WHAT do I need to do to feel good about myself spiritually?
- WHAT do I need to do to feel good about myself financially?
- WHAT do I need to do to feel good about myself socially?

- WHAT do I need to do to feel good about myself personally?
- WHAT do I need to do to feel good about myself professionally?
- WHAT would I like to do or be in one year?
- Five years?
- Twenty?

Set an appointment with yourself to sit down with a comforting cup of tea and spend time answering each of these questions. You owe that to yourself. When you have shaped the answers, you will be on your way to an exciting new future. Dream BIG. You will soon be living what you only thought were impossible dreams. Tap into the magic in you. Why the wait? **WHY THE WEIGHT? DARE TO BE GREAT!**

Then, read the next chapter, immediately. You'll be glad you did, because you will discover the POWER of...

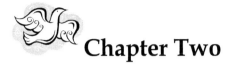 **Chapter Two**

The New You — Body, Mind and Spirit!

This can be YOUR year—your year of the new YOU—your year for you to change EVERYTHING. You can RESHAPE YOUR BODY, MIND AND SPIRIT! Take a few minutes to read this chapter, and change your life forever.

Think about it. If you could improve your life in any way, what would you like to make even better? Let yourself dare to dream...dare to dream about what COULD be different. Most people reading this book want to change PHYSICALLY, by shedding excess pounds. Now beyond just losing weight, what else would you like to transform? Imagine just a few small modifications that could take you to new levels, where you could be your best person you ever envisioned you could be—inside and out.

Remember, your weight can be the one thing that touches upon everything else. Your body, mind and spirit are all connected. Don't let those extra pounds stop you from achieving all your other dreams. Let go of any extra burden you carry, and you will be inspired to reach for your topmost dreams. You will continue to reach higher and higher to fulfill your heart's desires. You will find you are open to more things to keep on improving your life.

You may want to expand **INTELLECTUALLY**, as you take a new interest in untapped experiences. You might want to learn new languages, read fascinating books, or travel to new places.

What would you like to change **PERSONALLY**? Do you want more patience? A better sense of humor? A more positive outlook? Pick one thing you want to work on, and find three things each day to enhance that new trait.

You can explore a new life **SPIRITUALLY**. Are you aspiring to live your highest vision that was in the mind of God at your creation? Would you like to have a closer relationship with your Maker? Could you grow from more time spent in meditation or prayer? How could you move to a higher ground to live more abundantly in the love that is God?

You can change **SOCIALLY**. Like a Girl Scout, you can: "Make new friends, yet keep the old." Associate with winners. Find people who are examples of success. Surround yourself with people who ask more of you than you do yourself. Connect with people that you want as your role models. Think, walk and act as the person you wish to become. Perform your role, as if you are an actor or actress in a starring part, because you are. Know exactly what you want to become, and visualize it as part of you. Write your plan to achieve these goals and follow through with your appropriate steps to meet these people. Make new friends. Get more active friends in your life.

You can be the new you **FINANCIALLY**. Do you believe you could? Believing is achieving. Expect that every good and wonderful thing is now flowing into your life. Consistently deliver your best. Write your plan to achieve new goals to generate money. Do three things each day to make this happen.

You could become a new you **PROFESSIONALLY**.
You could take yourself to new heights and new jobs.
Think about all the fresh adventures you can put
into your life—if you will only dare to dream. PLEASE
dare to dream!

Shape a specific goal for each of your following areas:
**PHYSICAL, INTELLECTUAL, PERSONAL, SOCIAL,
PROFESSIONAL, FINANCIAL**, and **SPIRITUAL**. Then write
at least three benefits that you will receive if you attain each
of these goals. Next, follow through with your appropriate
action steps. Do three things each day to make all of these
things happen on every level.

You can do a lot of things to make this your best year, and
your best YOU, ever. You can make it all happen. It's up to
you. You can accomplish magnificent things. Take a look at
a calendar just three weeks from now. In three weeks' time,
if you really decided you could make a change, what do you
think you can accomplish? Close your eyes right now, and
think about what could be different? What kind of major
things could you make happen?

Let's start with pounds. Do a little quick math. You know
what you are capable of, especially if you are focused. How
much weight can you lose safely and realistically three
weeks from now—Six pounds? Eight? Ten? In three weeks
time you could possibly fit into a new clothing size—if you
say it, it will happen. It's all part of your whole mental
process. If you commit to your goal—if you proclaim your
goal—if you share your goal—if you tell other people about
your goal, it will come about. The universe is that way.

This is all part of what is known as ***POWER* LIVING**.
Use the ***POWER*** principles to be:

- *P ositive*
- *O pen*
- *W illing*
- *E nthusiastic*
- *R esponsible*

Taken together, the above recipe can help you reach your life's ultimate potential. In case you think the **POWER Principles** sound too good to be true, know that I have actually been conservative in my claim. In reality, if you use the formula—you will take charge of your life.

The **POWER** Principles propelled me to lose sixty pounds and to launch me into the career and life of my dreams. **POWER** is the magic within each of us. Our population is ripe for this book on **POWER LIVING**, and will be for many years to come. Sixty-two percent of all Americans (97 million people) are overweight or obese, and don't know WHY. Worse yet, they don't know HOW to do anything about it. People need an easy method to lose weight, and this book allows them to do so in a hurry.

By picking up this book, Dear Reader, you have demonstrated that you have responsibility (one of the **SEVEN KEYS TO SKINNY PEOPLE,** a special chapter which is covered later in this book). In other words, you are able to respond, and make things happen. After all, there are three types of people in this world:

1. **Those who MAKE things happen.**
2. **Those who WATCH things happen.**
3. **And those who wonder: *WHAT HAPPENED?***

Which one are you? Be the type who MAKES things happen. You can make MAGIC happen, if you allow yourself to seek your potential. Take a look at some things that could make a difference in your life. Close your eyes for a moment and think:

> • ***What will make me feel like a winner?***
> (Create a detailed dream that conjures up specific pictures and emotions.)

- ***How do I want to see myself in three weeks? In three months? A year?*** In just a short amount of time you could see a total difference. The weeks, months and years go by anyway. Why not make them count?

A GOAL IS A DAYDREAM WITH A DEADLINE

Do you have daydreams like this? *"Someday I'm going to get skinny. Someday I'm going to get a different job...someday I'm going to go to Europe...**someday**..."* But somehow, someday never comes. A goal is a target or aspiration combined with a plan to meet that objective. A <u>goal</u> has a deadline. A <u>dream</u> seldom does.

What do you want to achieve in your precious lifetime? What kind of a person do you wish to become? What personality traits do you want to acquire? Who are you and what are you meant to do with your God-given gifts? Where do you want to go? What would you like to be doing as your life's work? What kind of people would you like for your closest friends?

These questions are your most important questions you will ever answer. Only YOU know your answers. Reach high for your uppermost wishes. Write them all down. Seeing your goals in writing becomes part of your promise to follow through. Next, write small steps you will take daily to achieve them. Then give yourself small deadlines along your way. ***"By the inch it's a cinch!"***

Remember the old Chinese proverb: "The journey of a thousand miles begins with a single step." You will take that single step today when you sit down and write your goals and your daily steps you will take to achieve them.

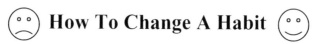

How To Change A Habit

It takes twenty-one days to change a habit. We are all creatures of habit. Everyone knows how hard it is to get rid of a bad habit. Habits control us without our even thinking about them. Some habits are healthy and some are unhealthy. Our bad habits are often developed when we are very young and have power over us until we take notice and take charge. People struggle to keep their old self-defeating habits because that is all they know. Often they live from the past, still using thoughts that limit them, from events that no longer serve them. They are not conscious of their possibilities because they are not open to change.

A habit is done automatically and instinctively without awareness. You put on the same shoe first each day. You eat with your same hand. You take the same route through the grocery store. Habits are made through repetition. You are the architect of your life. You can improve your life, as you improve your body, mind and spirit.

You cannot change a habit by just thinking you will get rid of it, but you can create a new habit in its place. Taking a series of small steps in the right direction is your way to shape a new habit. Habits are not easy to break because people are creatures of comfort even in their misery. Your wish to change must be stronger than your need to keep your old behavior. In order for change to happen, you have to want something like you would want water in the desert. Your first small step can be uncomfortable, yet it gets easier and easier, until finally it becomes difficult to go back to your old behavior.

☺ SMILES METHOD
6 Small Steps To Change:

1. **S ELECT** inspiring goals that are exciting enough to ignite your passions.
2. **M ARK** measurable milestone that will happen in three weeks time.
3. **I DENTIFY** what you are doing now that DOES NOT WORK.
4. **L IST** three action steps you will take daily, starting now.
5. **E NVISION** the magnificent benefits you gain at the end.
6. **S ET** a date for accomplishment and sign.

Soon new habits will become a part of you and your old habits will no longer exist. Remember every small step you take is never lost. If you fall off your horse, just get right back on again. Don't beat yourself up or the horse, either. Many people figure if they blew it for one meal, then the whole day is shot. Any progress you have made is still waiting for you to take your next step. Get rid of any *all or none* thinking, which often defeats people. If you lose a dollar does that mean you should throw away your wallet?

Set yourself up to win. For instance, carry a snack-attack survival kit with you at all times. Don't go to risky places or hang out with risky people who will tempt you until you are strong. Get rid of the wrong kind of foods and put the right kind in your shopping cart and refrigerator.

Repetition is a powerful tool for change. Listening to positive affirmations on audiotapes energizes you to reprogram your subconscious mind with your new thoughts and ideas you are trying to incorporate into your life.

First of all, what benefits could you gain, if you were to achieve your weight loss milestone in three weeks? We're talking return on time invested. What would you get out of your efforts? To answer this question, let's eavesdrop on a workshop I held in California:

> *Joanne: I'm looking forward to the confidence I'll gain. If I reach my goal then I'll be able to do a lot of other things. I'll be more able to reach for setting up my own business, and creating new customers.*

> *Margie: I'm picturing what it will be like to be able to bend over and tie my shoes without effort. That would really mean a difference to me.*

> *Brenda: I'm going to fit into the smaller clothes in my own closet. That will make me feel terrific.*

By the way, I want to encourage you always to fit into your next smallest size that you can possibly find right now. Don't allow yourself to wear anything that is too large. When you suck it in, and tuck it in—when you make yourself feel skinnier—you ARE skinnier, and you look at least five pounds thinner. So keep on trying to slip into smaller clothes, and don't wait until the end of your journey until you buy a new outfit. A lot of people do, and they wear the same old loosey-goosey muumuus. Those loose outfits give a lot of permission, and a chance to slide backwards.

> *Louise: My self-esteem will improve. Everyone will see the change in me.*

Self-esteem. Can that make the difference when you've still got a ways to go?

> *Louise: You bet! I may not be done in three weeks time, but it will be such an encouragement to me to keep going.*

> *Bobbie: My health is going to improve. I will have more energy. I'm going to be having knee surgery, so I want to go into that operation weighing less, and I know my recovery time will be much faster.*

Let me share with you at this time that I too am going in for an operation. I need a total hip replacement, and the reason I need it is because I have osteo-arthritis. My doctor told me that I probably did some damage to myself when I was carrying all my extra weight all those years. So, I want to commend you, those of you who are doing what needs to be done to lose your excess weight now. If you have a health issue with possible surgery ahead of you, you'll be encouraged by what my doctor said to me. He said: "Thank goodness you've lost all that weight first, because your recovery is going to be so much easier and so much better!"

Weight is often centered in our heads. If we can address that gray matter, right between our two ears, that's where our fat really is. We need to tell ourselves we can do it, and then DO IT! Our health could most definitely be improved, if we lose our excess weight. We will see other magnificent things, as well.

> *Janet: I have high blood pressure, and I'm going to make an appointment with my doctor soon, to see if he can't take me off of my cholesterol and high blood pressure medications, now that I'm losing weight.*

Your doctor will love you. I'll be willing to bet that there will be a difference with your cholesterol and blood pressure numbers, and you might even be able to get rid of those old pills. They slow you down, and often cause water retention. It's such a double battle. You'll be so glad when you're off of them. For me, twelve years of high blood pressure medication, are now gone. Of course, you will want to work with your doctor. Don't go off of them on your own.

What are some other benefits?

> *Marilyn: I'm going to feel comfortable in an airline seat this summer when I visit my grandchildren.*

> *Sandy: I'm going to be able to cut my toenails.*

> *Darlene: ...and polish them.*

Susan: I'm going to look good in a bathing suit.

That's great, Susan. Now, take that one step further. Picture a color, a size and a style. Try to be very specific.

Susan: I'm seeing a pink bikini in a size eight.

Wonderful! The sharper your vision of your goal, the more likely you are to achieve it. By the way, you do have the right, you know, to "bare arms." You also have your right to bare legs. There's no reason why you can't do that now. Love yourself all the way.

So, you can wear shorts, you can wear bathing suits, you can get into those size eight's. However, you have got to give up some things in order to do other things. There are going to be some obstacles in your way. What are you going to have to give up? I'd like to tell you how I overcame my most difficult hurdle when I was on my journey.

One of my problems occurred every time I went to my bridge club. The ladies served wonderful goodies—chips, dip, fudge, brownies, pizza. There I was trying to lose weight, and yet every time I went, I'd be facedown in the cheese balls. So, I had to decide, should I give up bridge? No! I most certainly couldn't give up bridge. Yet I could give up the tempting munchies, by substituting something else.

So I would say to the hostess, "Do you mind, I've brought these along to share?" And in a Tupperware container I'd have cherry tomatoes, carrots, celery, and other things.

The hostess would always say, "Of course." She may not have known I had to do that for my own survival. Yet I knew if I didn't, I'd give in to those decadent munchies.

What are some things you know you'll have to give up, in order to see the changes you wish to see in three weeks?

Barbara: I'm trading sleeping in for exercise.

Now, that is a great habit to adopt. Put first things first—you and your exercise. An effective loser knows that's important. You know how to prioritize. Ask yourself: where have my priorities been misaligned? Where am I losing out on myself? Perhaps your priority has been to have an immaculate house. Maybe that doesn't have to be a priority. Maybe you can give less time to your house, and a little more time to you. How about your in-basket? Does it always have to get emptied? If you re-prioritize, maybe you can give yourself some time to exercise.

Bert: I'm going to give up my late-night TV.

That is very wise, because if you stay up for late-night TV, you will have too much downtime, and you won't have enough uptime. However, by getting started early in your morning you'll have more energy, plus you'll start a lifetime change. It takes three weeks to change a habit. If you start doing that, it could change your life. It could even change the length of your life. Wow! Think about that.

> *Jessie: I'm going to give up ice cream. I decided that it's not worth it for 5 minutes of pleasure. All these weeks I've been working so hard to take off weight. I'm going to say: **"A moment on your lips, forever on your hips,"** and post that on my refrigerator.*

Another one to keep in mind is: **"Nothing tastes as good as thin feels!"** You are wise to limit those trigger foods, because they awaken the "crazies" in us. They wake up our adrenalin, and one always means more. In fact, one often means four. For you, it's ice cream. Substituting a low fat yogurt might be an idea. For many it's chocolate. If you know your red light foods, you realize you can only handle just a bit. In fact, for me, it is nuts. I can't handle them. I know and I recognize that. I could never have a whole bowl sitting next to me. If you realize your sabotage food, you are closer to having it under control. Even white bread can be a trigger. It's far safer to have breads with wheat or fiber.

> *Peggy: I'm finding I need to work on instant gratification. If I can wait five minutes—if I can just postpone my eating, I feel more in control.*

That's a problem that starts when we are kids. If we fall down and hurt our knee, our Mom gives us a cookie. Instant gratification. An instant band-aid, and the band-aid Is imbred into us from the beginning, in the form of food. If we feel bad, our answer is food. Try to spot that pattern.

Now, in order to see the changes you hope to see in three weeks, you have to make a few changes. So, what is one change that you will commit to this week?

> *Jerry: I plan to shop and have lots of healthy snacks on hand. Things that are easy to grab, like cherry tomatoes, and grapes.*

> *Sandy: I plan to make plenty of vegetable soup. I always see a big weight loss when I do. It fills me and satisfies me. My family loves it, too. In fact, lately, I've been adding jalapenos, and it's great.*

> *Dotty: I'm going to use controlled portions this week. I plan to get out my measuring cups and spoons and stop being a "Pinocchio" about how much I'm eating.*

> *Vera: I'm going to <u>BYOV</u>, bring my own veggie dish to share at a potluck I'm going to this weekend.*

That could be a big change to make for the rest of your life. If you bring your own dish to share to every event you go to, you will rarely succumb to pizza, fried chicken, fudge, and things that would get you off-track. I could never have made my goal without that strategy: BYOV. I was a slow-learner. I only lost a pound a week, yet I could have lost all the faster. I would undo all my hard work every week when I was at yet another gathering with tempting foods. Start doing that now, and you'll see an easier, faster journey.

> *Jan: I'm going to set my alarm fifteen minutes earlier and get up and walk.*

That will boost your metabolism. Make yourself a morning person, and you'll burn more calories. Do what works, and stop doing what doesn't work. Doing what works is about choosing to do only those things, which produce the results you desire. It is important to think, feel, envision and speak only what you wish to experience. Visualize yourself as being, doing and having what you need right now.

Here's an example of a **SMILES** **METHOD** contract:

SIX SMALL STEPS TO CHANGE.

What would you like to improve *PHYSICALLY?*

1. **S ELECT** inspiring GOALS to ignite your passions:
   - *I want to lose twenty pounds.*
   - *I want a flatter tummy.*
   - *I want to look good in a bathing suit.*
   - *I want shapely, toned arms.*
   - *I want to get off medications.*
2. **M ARK** measurable MILESTONES in three weeks: (Remember, it takes three weeks to form a new habit.)
   - *I get up without hitting the snooze button.*
   - *I tighten my belt another notch.*
   - *I feel greater energy and ease in doing things.*
   - *I make healthier food choices.*
3. **I DENTIFY** what you do that DOESN'T WORK:
   - *I get up too late to exercise.*
   - *I spend too much time watching TV.*
   - *I avoid eating vegetables and fruits.*
   - *I choose fried, fatty or unhealthy foods.*

4. L IST three ACTION steps you will take daily:
- *I set the alarm clock a half-hour earlier.*
- *I bring home only healthy food choices.*
- *I limit my TV watching, and do more activity.*
- *I eat five to nine servings of fruits/vegetables.*

5. E NVISION the BENEFITS you gain at the end:
- *I feel more self-confidence.*
- *I experience better health.*
- *I look great in a size eight bikini!*
- *I now can reach all my other goals, as well.*

6. S ET a DATE of accomplishment: *(For a sensible weight-loss, strive for one to two and a half pounds per week after your initial water loss which occurs in your first week)*
- *Date_____*
- *Your signature. (This makes it a commitment.)*

Now complete contracts in order to reshape all areas of your life: **PHYSICALLY, INTELLECTUALLY, SPIRITUALLY, SOCIALLY, FINANCIALLY, PROFESSIONALLY AND PERSONALLY.**

Your goals can become reality, if you let them. Make contracts like the example above. Carry them in your purse or briefcase and review them throughout your day. Time you spend in doing this assignment will be your best investment you have ever made in yourself. You are about to reshape your body, mind and spirit. Your results can be life changing, as promised. Read on and see.

The following chapter is an adapted transcript from a support group meeting led by the author.

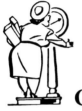

Chapter Three

The Final Insult

Did you ever stare at a photo and wonder WHO is that FAT person, only to discover the person is YOU? Did you ever announce to yourself, "This is the last straw!" Did you ever hear your own commanding voice say to you, "Enough, already—I have got to lose some weight!"

It is called your "defining" moment—a split-second decision that comes from a final insult. It occurs in the matter of a single second where you can no longer zip up your pants, or the instant you simply refuse to buy a bigger size. Perhaps it is in seeing a video of you that surprises and insults you, or a kid who says: "Mommy, WHY is that lady FAT?" Perhaps someone asks if you are pregnant. That moment is for-all-time a flash you remember vividly. It is that split second that you make up your mind and say to yourself, "I guess I am ready to do something about this problem."

My moment came when I saw a photo of my mother. That is, I THOUGHT it was my mother, but afterward I recognized it was a picture of ME! For a year prior to that picture, I stopped weighing myself. I found I weighed as much as my husband, so I simply went into denial.

But when I realized I was the one in that photograph, it was an inconceivable shock. I knew I had been "fluffing" up, but I thought I could hide that fact under the muumuus I wore. The image I saw made me recognize what the whole world knew all along—what I thought was my own little secret.

To my horror, I looked just like my mother when she died. That meant I looked twenty years OLDER than I should be. As much as I loved my mother, she was NOT my ideal role model. She was exceedingly overweight when she died, and it was agonizing to realize I was going down the same path. No doubt one day, I would be going to an early grave, as well. The feeling was panic—it was fear—it was repulsion.

 I'm sure many of you may recall an incident when you had to lie on your bed to zip up your jeans, or you could not bend over to tie your shoes, or maybe you had to have somebody help you get unzipped, and it was a humbling experience. Remember that Kodak moment? Capture the way you looked, the way you felt, and what came out of it. Shut your eyes and experience this once again. Ugh!

It is a crisp picture—a snapshot in history—like man's first walk on the moon. If you were alive then, you remember that moment vividly, even now. You can describe where you were, the people around you, the feelings you felt.

Remember your own historical event. Whatever that peak experience was, value your "defining" moment—your last-straw incident that brought you to comprehend it was time to do something. That memory can strengthen you, and work as a magnificent fixation, along with your feeling that grew out of it, whether it was disgust, horror, queasiness, embarrassment, disappointment or???

Sharon: I was shopping for what I thought was my size. I took a bunch of clothes into the dressing room, and I could not get any of them on, no matter what I did. I swore I would not allow myself to buy the next size, because I just knew that would lead to the next size after that.

Adrienne: I'll never forget an excruciating experience I had at a theatre. I became wedged into those narrow seats, and I got stuck. I was horrendously embarrassed. I needed help to get me unstuck! To make matters worse, I was in terrible agony the next day with black and blue marks and bruises all over. It was my wake-up call, a powerful incident, and I knew something had to be done.

Tiffany: I was at the mall, just walking along, and I saw a woman's reflection in a shop window. She was really fat. I thought, "Oh, my goodness, she looks so aged and dreary."...And then I saw it was ME! Until that moment, I imagined I was still at my twenty-five-year-old figure of one-hundred-twenty-pounds. It just dawned on me how I didn't even recognize myself. I was mortified!

Sarah: After each baby, I ballooned to the next larger size, and the next, and the next. Finally, I graduated to a mass I never thought I could allow myself to become ever in my lifetime. I refused to buy anything. That was a drop-dead moment. It was staring me in the face, and it really scared me. I kept scaring myself with what would happen to me in five years? In ten years?

Dr. Elly: After I sat and sat and munched dry-roasted nuts and drank red wine while completing my doctoral dissertation, I ran into a gentleman I hadn't seen in awhile, from Las Vegas. He used to pick me up in Los Angeles and we drove to school. We were both in a PhD. Program, back then. "Whatever happened to you?" he questioned. That did it for me— the reality check of how I had been neglecting myself. I subsequently lost 40+ pounds.

Bob: My shock happened at my annual physical. My doctor told me it was time to get worried. My high blood pressure and cholesterol levels were spiking. He advised me to do something fast, or I wasn't going to live much longer. It was as plain and frightful as that.

If you remember a feeling that came out of your moment, do something with that emotion. Capture and use it. Some of those defining moments can insult you, terribly. Hang onto those instants, and your feelings that came out of them. Revisit and go back to other chapters. You can trace your patterns, and see how you got to that final "fluffy" you. This awareness will kick-start your discovering of old destructive habits. You may also be grateful for new and beautiful feelings of self-love and self-acceptance.

Check Other Chapters

What habits helped you to get to your defining moment? What were your crucial decisions along your way? My weight was never a problem in grade school or high school. In fact, my mother called me "snake ribs" because I consumed large amounts of almost any food, and it would go right through me like a snake.

But then came college days. Anyone who has ever been to Madison, Wisconsin most likely remembers good old State Street. Have you ever heard of "freshman fifteen?" That is what happens the first year or so to kids who go off to college. They are exposed to lots of freedom and new choices. They are faced with options, such as what to eat in the school cafeteria. There is dorm food and fast food, and drinking and partying, and a whole new atmosphere.

In Wisconsin, the drinking age was eighteen years. Up and down State Street were all kinds of bars, and we were welcome! I found out quickly how beer could bloat me.

After college, I joined a great partying faculty. Being a new teacher, I tried to keep up with the rest who would party in that cold weather—just to stay warm. There were a lot of TGIF's—Thank God It's Friday nights. That meant two-for-one "Harvey Wallbangers." Well, one thing I didn't know then is—every jigger of liquor means a lot of calories...and a drink like that is not just one jigger, but in all probability three. Then they started with TGIW's—Thank God It's Wednesday nights, with two-for-one "Rusty Nails." (You wouldn't even want to know the calories in some of those drinks, but of course, you needed to eat more, so you could stay sober. That packed on the pounds!)

Go back and revisit YOUR life's chapters. When did your weight gain start? Maybe you could testify, yes—marriage packed on the pounds. I married my prince charming, and soon I got a chubby hubby. Instantly, both of us gained ten pounds, twenty pounds together. What partners we were.

We received a couple of wedding gifts we should never have opened, because they began the next era of more fat and more pounds. One of those gifts was a deep-fat fryer. I battered and deep-fried chicken, French fries, onion rings, shrimp, and even donuts. You name it. Little did I know then—fried foods were on the top of the list when it comes to fat. (Now, I have new habits of eating things that are baked, broiled, or grilled, without the skin or the batter.) I would highly recommend to any newly married bride, or otherwise, to give back the deep fryer. Don't even open it. Or, use it as a planter. It makes a great conversation piece!

An additional gift we received was an electric frying pan. I used it, (as my mother always did), to fry a pound of bacon. Then I cooked the eggs right on top of the grease. Yum! Another Wisconsin favorite I made for my husband was beef stroganoff. All the beef and cream was doubtless the start of my cholesterol and high blood pressure problem that showed up in later years. So...watch out for fried food. It means plaque in your veins!

I found having kids helps pack on the pounds, too. We had two darling children, a boy and a girl, who are now adults. Being the good Mommy, I coaxed them to eat everything. Of course, if they didn't eat it all—you know who did. I was a member of the "clean plate club." I can still hear about the poor starving children in China. My mother always said: "Eat your plate!"

Here's a news update—the starving children in China are now getting fat. Perhaps we all replay those mental tapes from our mothers, but you can now get rid of your guilt. Write that one off. It's no longer an excuse! Instead, try a new thought, because, otherwise, YOU become the human waste machine. The food you are trying to stop from wasting goes down your own waste disposal. It goes to "waist," instead! Next time you hear those old tapes say to you: "Waste Not." substitute the new spelling: w-a-i-s-t.

> *Arlene: My husband used to accuse me of always wasting good food for which he had to pay. Now, I find he is adopting some of the same healthy thinking I recently introduced. He actually leaves a bite or two on his plate. It is such a feeling of freedom for me, because I feel as though I have been given permission to leave that food behind.*

What a tremendous bravo for both of you. If you can say, "I'm in control...the food is not in control of me...I don't need to eat every single last bite"—you have graduated to a new level of self-love.

> *Janet: I serve myself much smaller portions, these days. If I eat out, I ask for the senior menu, or I order appetizers.*

Another strategy is to ask for an EARLY "doggie bag." If you ask for it when your meal comes, you can put half of your food away for another meal, right then and there. If you wait and ask later, however, you're likely to eat all but a few bites, feel foolish, and finish your whole meal, anyway.

Don't' worry. Restaurants do not consider your request tacky in the least. In fact, a survey conducted at some of the most exclusive restaurants in Orange County showed sixty percent of the patrons asked for a take-home container.

Help yourself, rather than sabotage yourself. Often, you do the right thing by picking the right portion, and choosing the healthy choice. The trouble begins later, as you clear the table. That's where my own self-destruction emerges.

I cannot handle putting away leftovers. I find myself nibbling and snibbling, even if I'm full. One day I asked my husband for support. To my amazement, I found he was completely willing to take on the job of scraping the plates. I learned all I had to do was A-S-K in order to G-E-T. Occasionally, I remind him because he forgets how important this is to me. To my astonishment I find once again—all I have to do is ask. This is something Dr. Elly wrote in putting into force the strategies of *The Good Girl Syndrome* in her book by the same name.

> *Sarah: I, too, have found that my whole family will chip in and help clear the table if I tell them why it is so important to me. But sometimes, I even do something to destroy the leftovers, like pour salt or sugar all over it.*

That's one more excellent example of control. A further exercise is to choose the thing you crave the most. Pick a food you have a hard time saying "no," to, like a piece of chocolate cake or pizza. Turn on the water, hold it in your hand, and watch it dissolve down the drain. A strange transformation will start to happen within you, as you write over the top of those tapes in your head that say: "waste not." I strongly recommend you try this practice at least once or twice, just to show yourself you can take command.

But we were talking about chapters along the way that caused us to reach our "fluffy" state from which we are trying to move away. One of my own episodes included a time when I was down-and-out. I was diagnosed with cancer of the kidney and I had to have the bad kidney removed. After the surgery, I became extremely weak and sedentary. Just getting out of bed was a challenge. Eventually, I was able to walk, yet my fragile state became my excuse for my not exercising, and the medication caused extreme water retention. Between the two, I gained an additional ten pounds.

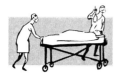 If you had surgery, or a serious injury, or need to take any type of medication causing fluid retention, you will find your journey to losing weight is much harder. The water retention and lack of activity may cause you extra pounds. If you have these problems, I have all the respect in the world for you, yet it can be done. You can still lose weight. Read these inspirational stories:

> *Pam: After breast cancer, I gained twenty-five pounds from medication and chemotherapy. My sister said she had a friend who was able to lose the "after-cancer" weight with healthy diet and exercise. I've been trying that too, and I've almost lost those twenty-five pounds.*

> *Madeleine: I am diabetic, and my medication has bloated me enormously. However, since coming to your classes, I found the right kinds of fruits, veggies and fiber, along with my daily walking regimen, have contributed to my forty-pound weight loss.*

> *Betty: My doctor has me on hormones, which puff me up, immensely. Nonetheless, I am happy to say, I have again found my prior figure by making healthy choices.*

So, you can do it! It's a lot harder, but it can be done. Be determined! By the way, some of those medications have less fluid retention than others. Always ask both your doctor and your pharmacist if there is another alternative. Often your pharmacist has more information on the latest drugs, and if he/she has a suggestion, go back to your doctor and ask if that could be a suitable choice for you. (Be sure to check my chapter in this book entitled: HOW TO

EAT MORE, YET WEIGH LESS to find the foods referred to by Madeleine, Betty and Pam.)

A different time in my life, which resulted in weight gain, was when I was sorely in need of comfort. There was a huge, black period in my life when I lost my Mom, my Dad and all three of my brothers. So many dear family members, so important in my life were dead! Suddenly, I felt lost and empty. I turned to food to soothe me. Food was my drug of choice. It was my comforter, yet it became my sabotage.

A lot of us are comfort eaters. We go to food for consolation. Become aware of that. Don't think food will bring happiness. It's like a nasty Halloween Trick! Instead, try non-sabotage, non-food rewards when you need to have enticements. Become aware you are just stuffing down emotions when you reach for food. It is substituting sweets for emotional satisfaction or even sex.

Instead, get those emotions out—talk to a friend, get some exercise, get things that are pampering to you. Food is not your true comfort. It will not make you happy. Be gentle with yourself, yet don't indulge yourself with food. Try the best therapy of all—retail therapy. Shop for some treat, other than food that will make you feel really good. Close your eyes and think of what you will do for you!

Today your assignment is to find your most insulting picture you can find of yourself. Put it on your refrigerator. That image is what you want to move AWAY from. Put it side-by-side with a picture of the "you" that you want to look like, the one you want to move TOWARD.

Get a Role Model

If you don't have a prior picture of your ideal body image, then do what I did. Since I was never as thin as I envisioned as my goal, there were no prior photos from which to choose. That didn't stop me. I found an early picture of Lauren Bacall, my idol since childhood, and pasted my face right on top of hers. I looked so classy in her fabulous clothes and figure!

She was my role model since I was a five-year-old, playing with my treasured set of Lauren Bacall paper-dolls. Now I was playing again, yet this time for a more serious purpose. I was aspiring to capture her energy and longevity, knowing she was still gorgeous and shapely in her seventies.. That clipping, along with my own "fat-lady" photo, looked at me each time I opened my refrigerator. For the entire year while I was trying to lose my sixty pounds, I deliberated which of the two images I wanted to look like most before I decided to eat anything. That time to hesitate and consider helped me immeasurably.

Next, I created a role-model scrapbook of all the people I admired for one attribute or another. I collected pictures of stars and celebrities who influenced me in my life. I imagined what it would be like to look and feel as good as they must feel.

Julie Andrews made some astounding life-changing movies. I had grown up with her examples of incredible wholesomeness, health and energy in movies such as **Mary Poppins,** and **The Sound of Music.** I was energized when I thought of how young she still appears today. It helped convince me I could be a winner and take control of my weight.

Richard Simmons helped me to reshape my body, mind and spirit. His poignant honesty and sincerity in his books like **Never Give up,** and his fun loving exercise in **Sweatin' to the Oldies,** gave me the lift, and inspiration I needed to continue.

I thought about the beautiful Barbara Streisand singing **People**. The lyrics: *"People who love people are the luckiest people in the world"* struck me because those people learn to love themselves first. I needed to start loving myself, more. Doesn't everyone need this lesson?

Angela Lansbury helped me to bring balance to my life. Her fit and lively portrayal in **Murder She Wrote,** served as a breath of confirmation to me that I could be healthy like her. Her poignant candor and wit in her biography, **Balancing Act,** empowered me to believe in the magic of believing in myself.

Sophia Loren was another positive influence upon me. Her age-defying beauty and grace always astounded me. I found her cookbook with healthy Italian gourmet recipes, and thought—no wonder she looks like she does! She cooks with wonderful combinations of eggplant and mushrooms, rice with turkey, chestnuts and dried fruit. Many of her recipes are meatless. This inspired me to cook with more vegetables like she did, and off came the pounds.

What Would My Role Model Do?

Whenever I was faced with a food temptation, I asked myself what my heroes or heroines would do in a given situation. When I went to a cocktail party, I visualized myself making the same slim choices the incomparable Bo Derek would select if she were approaching the buffet table, instead of me.

When I was tempted to press the snooze alarm and skip my morning exercise routine, I pictured Richard Simmons jumping happily out of bed, to do a fun routine in his cheerful workout outfits.

When I grew tired of the same diet and fitness routine, I projected what I might look like at Jack LaLanne's age. Would I have his energy? His wit? Would I even be able to attract a man? Or would I grow old, fat and pathetic? Or be long dead?

Perky Julia Roberts is always a class act, ever effervescent and alluring. Would she wear my frumpy, figure-forgiving tunics and stretchy waistbands, or would she choose belts to tuck-in and suck-in her tummy? (By the way, I always found I looked an automatic five pounds thinner, if I tucked in my blouses and sucked in my tummy.)

Would Vanna White have a second helping of cheesecake? No, she would fill her tummy with vegetables first.

Would Connie Selleca eat a cheeseburger and super-sized fries? Never!

Would Barbara Streisand beat herself up with negative self-talk? Of course not!

I would make-believe I was one of those celebrities, and my habits gradually began to change. I experienced the results I so desired. I was losing weight!

Now, search for heroes of your own to use as role models. Make a list of all the things you admire about them. Begin to practice and incorporate their positive qualities in your daily routine. Go back to your defining moment. Experience the feelings. Capture your feelings. List those feelings. Write about them. Write about all the aspects of your life you want to change. Picture all the benefits and good feelings you will receive when you achieve that change.

Finally, search out the worst photo of yourself that you can find. Know there is something in the power of your most dreadful and abysmal recollections that will strengthen you because you have learned from it. Whatever that moment was, it was the best thing that ever happened to you, because you know you are never going back there again.

You are new today. You are the changed you. You are all those wonderful qualities. You are the greatest **YOU**!

Be sure to read the next chapter where you will learn to never take anything **PERSONALLY** again, because you will make...

The following chapter is an adapted transcript from a workshop led by the author.

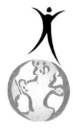

Chapter Four

Four Agreements
Will Change Your World

A.gree.ment (a-'gre-ment) **noun. 1.** Arrangement as to course of action.

If you make THE FOUR AGREEMENTS in this chapter, your life will change. I promise. You will reshape your body, mind and spirit, and you will be "power living."

Recently, I had the experience of attending a workshop given by Don Miguel Ruiz, who wrote the book, *The Four Agreements*. He is a wise Toltec, with a philosophy going back to basic truths of ancient wisdom. Oprah Winfrey says reading his book changed her life. It has already been published in twenty-two different languages, and has sold well over-a-million copies. You may have read the book, or you are familiar with its content—in which case, you can most likely see how it ties-in perfectly with weight-loss. It is about the power of the mind—something for which we are all striving. Don Miguel transformed many people's lives, and he positively influenced mine.

Don Miguel concluded his talk that afternoon with one key idea—to go out and teach **The Four Agreements** to everyone. I was struck with the idea teaching **The Four Agreements** would be a powerful message in my lectures on weight-loss, and to include in this book, as well. Afterward, I stayed to speak with him, and asked for his input. I told him I was helping people change their lives on all levels, starting with the need to change physically, and lose weight. He said the problem of weight-gain was a natural place to incorporate his teachings, and he gave me his full approval.

I was excited and I began to teach his philosophy to my weight-loss support-groups that week, and found **The Four Agreements** were greatly received...and so, dear reader, I am also sharing with you the wisdom taught me by Don Miguel Ruiz. This chapter is an adapted transcript from a support-group meeting in Southern California.

The Four Agreements is a book with a philosophy that gets into your head, and makes you take a look at rewriting some of your old "tapes" in your head, so you become more positive. The book questions many things, which are lies. In fact, many of the chatterings in your mind are lies— different things people have told you—voices you heard when you were little. As a result, you believed them, and you continue to tell yourself the same negative things.

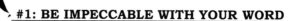

#1: BE IMPECCABLE WITH YOUR WORD

Your first agreement to your journey of power is: BE IMPECCABLE WITH YOUR WORD. Your IMPECCABLE WORD refers to words you tell others, as well as language you tell yourself within, (also known as Positive Self-Talk). You have a whole world of recordings in your mind from different people who have said things to you through the years. Diverse voices you hear have left an imprint on you in one way or another. Some memories make you feel good about yourself—other recollections make you feel bad. You allow the disapprovals to come back at you and haunt you. Those internal mumblings are like snakes. Don Miguel refers to your mind as a *mitote,* where the voices of a thousand influences talk at once, and no one understands the other.

Sometime during the mid-1980's, a study was done which you may recall. I remember the experiment well, because my son was in fourth-grade, and my daughter in the sixth-grade. The research involved a group of severely retarded children. They were isolated and taught by a group of teachers who were told to treat the youngsters as though they were geniuses. The teachers gave the kids the message they were exceptionally gifted. As you may guess, the children's self-esteem grew with these positive strokes. At the end of the study, their IQ's were re-tested. Each had advanced to an unprecedented intellectual level.

Well, the study made quite an impression on me. I thought about it, and wondered if the same principles might work on our children. Our son was in fourth grade at the time. He was getting B's and C's. My husband and I started giving him positive messages about how special he was, how one day he was going to do great things, and how he was going to excel because he had extraordinary gifts. I do not know how to explain this...but fifth grade was much better. In sixth grade, he got A's. From then on, he received all A's. In high school, he achieved a 4.0. In College he was one of the brightest in his class. He is up in San Jose, now starting a new company.

We spoke the same affirmative messages to our daughter, who was two years older. School was more difficult for her. I suspect some lies—some negative experiences damaged her self-esteem and kept playing in her head—where she could not accept or believe such praise. Ultimately, when she became an adult, and came to realize her authentic self, and focus on the dreams she wanted for her life—she went on to excel and do great things, as well. She graduated in the top 5% of her class, and is now a Registered Nutritionist, supervising her own center. My husband and I believe those words of encouragement made a difference in both of our children's lives.

You can see where messages from your past can come back at you, in your weight-loss situation, and are still haunting you. People may have told you lies you remember from when you were young. Perhaps somebody even said you were fat, or you had large thighs, or perhaps some sales clerk insulted you when you tried on something, which did not fit right. Something may still be hurting, continuing to bite like a rattlesnake. You need to be a warrior, and chop-off its ugly head, and kill it once-and-for-all.

I will never forget the sales lady who told me: "In order to hide your flaws, 'Dearie,' you need to look at the bathing-suits in this section." She was referring to extra-large-sized swimsuits with dreadful camouflage-skirts, like my grandmother used to wear.

Her words caused my self-esteem to crumble, and to this day, I still have self-doubt whenever I try on swimwear. I continue to wonder if my "flaws" are showing.

If you ruminate old dialogue within, you want to rewrite the words. In fact, obliterate them. Since you can only entertain one thought at a time, replace an unconstructive notion with a positive one. You can blot out ideas, or say: "Cancel! Cancel!" and you will rid yourself of those old unhelpful voices, and language you put in your mind. Be more IMPECCABLE with negatives you allow to enter your head. Choose, instead, affirmations to help you. Do not let any of those old influences emerge again.

In addition, be careful of utterances coming out of your mouth, which may be hurtful to others, as well. Choose your language well, so you do not devastate anybody else. The power of your remarks can be far-reaching. You must be aware of the amazing influence your speech can have on other people.

The effect of your statement can be incredibly life giving, and can also be terribly devastating. Don Luis relates an example in his book about a woman who was an especially pleasant, and caring person. However, she came home from work one day with an excruciating headache. Her little girl, who loved to sing, was singing the way little girls do. Well, the mother was in such horrible pain, she yelled to her child: "Stop it! Your voice is ugly!" The power of her remark was demoralizing. The mother's remark killed something within the little girl, and she never sang again. You need to take a look at what it means to be impeccable with your word.

#2: DON'T TAKE ANYTHING PERSONALLY

Don't take anything personally. Most people who are overweight have an amazingly fragile self-image. When something or somebody hurts their feelings—what do they do? They eat! Often the reason they go to food is for comfort. It is because they take things personally. They do not realize they are eating their emotions, as well.

Re-examine your day, and ask yourself, especially if you fell off-track, if something was said to make you feel inadequate or caused you some self-doubt. (If you can admit to that, half your battle has been won, because it is about "getting real." If you don't get real about fat, you get real fat, right?)

You cannot allow yourself to take things personally. People sometimes do not even know what they do or say. Like the girl who never sang again—she took her mother's words personally. Yet her mother was coming from a different place. The mother had her own drama going on, and the little one was actually not the reason, at all. Nonetheless, the child took it all in, and let it harm her.

So take a look at the words you let destroy you, or sabotage you. Turn them around, and re-write them. Try to be honest about the situations causing you to eat, and say: "Hey, this is what is really going on..." Take time to analyze what is happening. Say to yourself: "Am I eating this because I am truly hungry, or did somebody hurt my feelings? Did something tick me off? Is something happening because I am fragile today? Am I harboring something within me?" Do you relate to that?

> *Joan: My boss is a real nitpicker. Any project I submit always starts with her saying, "You did a nice job, but..." I resent those words, if she asks me to change or re-do things. I feel hurt, and I know I eat over it.*

Your boss selected some words we should all examine. She said, "You did a nice job, BUT..." Joan, how would you feel if she said, "You did a nice job, AND..."

> *Joan: I think, for some reason, I would feel a whole lot better.*

You probably cannot remember the first part, which started as a compliment. However, her choice of "BUT" negated everything she said before that "BUT." Had she used the word "AND" her praise would have remained intact. Remember the same lesson when you speak, and also when you hear the "BUT" word—never take it personally, or dish it out. By the way, check for similar management tools in dealing with yourselves and others by reading Ken Blanchard's ***The One Minute Manager***. His book helped me to gain control of my life, and helped me lose the sixty pounds.

> *Barbara: I am determined I can lose weight by myself, and nobody else can do it for me. Yet my husband, who never had a weight problem in his life, wants to be my "food police," and he says things like, "You don't want that." I take his words personally, and it causes me to want to rebel and eat, just to show him.*

Thank you for your openness. You are wise to be able to recognize those feelings and evaluate them. Some people would call what you just described as support, and you all come from a different place. So, look at each-and-every eating episode, truthfully. Are you taking something personally? Are you eating over it? Can you discuss it with each other? Sometimes what you do to yourself can be upsetting because you take another's words personally, and, yet, the person who said them has no idea.

I used to have such self-doubt I would get upset or hurt if someone merely honked at me on the freeway. (And, of course, I would go home and eat over the incident.) I was so sensitive, I found all kinds of reasons to believe no one liked me. I also had negative and judgmental feelings about others.

The best thing about now, however, is few things bother me, or hurt my feelings. I think my weight-loss helped a lot, and my taking time to nurture myself and do some journaling, made for a huge personal and spiritual change. Each night, before I go to bed, I try to write five things I am grateful for during the day, a habit that changed me. I got the idea from a book my daughter gave me, *Simple Abundance,* by Sarah Ban Breathnach. It even caused me to dream differently. Try it; I think you will like it.

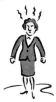

#3: DON'T MAKE ASSUMPTIONS

Don't ever make assumptions. You don't always know the answers. Find the courage to ask questions. Making assumptions can get you into a lot of trouble, and cause lost time, as well as weight-gain. Don't always take for granted you are communicating what you think you are, either. Avoid misunderstandings. With just this one agreement, you can completely transform your life and your weight.

When we feel hurt, depressed, and lonely, we often go to food for comfort. Yet the biggest assumption we could make is food will console us. Using food for comfort is the biggest lie and self-sabotage of all. If you are a comfort-eater, check your eating patterns for habits you will want to break.

Sometimes we turn to food because we suffer the loss of something or someone—a job, a boyfriend, or a promotion. It is all the same—we grieve a loss, just as we mourn a death. We try to heal ourselves with food.

I know, when I lost my five dear family members, I made the assumption I could fill that terrible, aching hole in my heart with food. Food was my friend. I stuffed down my grief, anger, loneliness, and even guilt for being alive. I quieted all those emotions with food. However, I found I could only fill my stomach—I could never fill my heart. What I actually needed was to fill myself with something else. I could either look at my glass as half-empty or half-full. I could assume my life was a bummer, or ask: "Why is it—I am the one who survived?"

When I started asking myself the above question, I started getting answers, which turned my feelings of despondency into expectancy. I got to believe in myself and that I was alive to achieve a higher purpose. I started setting goals for myself, and filling myself with encouraging declarations. The pounds magically peeled away, and a whole new life of promise emerged. I turned my profound loss into a powerful gain.

Another huge assumption we often make is people are talking about US. Frequently, we cause ourselves needless pain. I will never forget when I was a four-year-old child, lying in bed, listening to the conversation between my mother and my aunt, who were talking in the next room. I overheard them saying: "She's such a spoiled child." and: "She is such a little brat!"

I presumed they were talking about me. My little heart felt it would break. I cried myself to sleep that night. The next morning, I found they were making comments in reference to an article they read in the newspaper about some young royal princess.

Making assumptions people are talking about you may be something you did primarily in your childhood, but even recently, I overheard my husband talking on the phone. I thought I heard him say something like…"angry…? …No, she's not angry." Then he hung up. Feeling a bit miffed, I asked him why the other person imagined I was angry. Then he explained—they were not taking about me—but about someone else. How foolish to think I had fabricated something about **ME**! So I say, never presuppose it is about you. You will save yourself needless self-sabotage.

Making assumptions also gets us into trouble, and gets in the way of our weight-loss. Sometimes we think we know it all, and eat things we have no business eating, yet we have no clue as to how much fat or how many calories they contain. This supposition can spoil our progress. We can become a real "Pinocchio," and not even know it.

I used to believe I made an excellent choice at McDonald's, every time I chose the Filet-O-Fish. I figured fish was healthy, right? Wrong! Not if it is fried or battered. Besides, one sandwich was never enough. (Little did I know—white breads and fried-foods awakened my cravings.) For years, I understood chili rellenos were a wise choice in a Mexican restaurant. Only when I became "label-savvy" did I find out the truth. How does thirty-two grams of fat, and nine hundred calories, for a measly serving of two rellenos, strike you? I was dreadfully naïve.

I also found loads of salads, salad dressings and cheeses packed a big "fat punch." A mere two-tablespoons of Caesar dressing contain two-hundred-and-fifty calories. Even my eighty-five-year-old mother-in-law was of the mistaken notion—tuna fish salad was a prudent choice. Not so, we discovered. In fact, it is one of the unhealthiest things offered at a deli because of the mayonnaise. If it shines, it usually contains fat. Beware!

Also, have the courage to ask how something is prepared. Never take for granted the food is cooked in the healthiest manner—whether your spouse, a friend or a restaurant does the cooking. Even a broiled or grilled filet-of-fish is probably prepared with oil. Two tablespoons of light olive oil contain four hundred calories. If you ask ahead of time, you can always request "lite" or none. Be assertive when ordering. Don't speculate you can't "have it your way."

> *Martha: I was surprised to find restaurants are only too happy to accommodate my wishes. Now, I always ask for egg whites for my omelet, and I found I could substitute fruit or vegetables for other fattening side dishes. I used to be too intimidated to ever inquire if they would do such a thing.*

Good for you, Martha. Making assumptions in restaurants can get people into a lot of trouble, and cause lost time. They re-gain the weight they worked so hard to lose in the first place, to say nothing of the needless frustration endured from "yo-yo-ing" up and down on the scale. Don't always take for granted you are communicating what you think you are, either. Paraphrase, to make sure. Be assertive. Avoid misunderstandings.

> *Sally: I was misinformed for years. I thought the green kale or parsley on the plate was a decoration. I never ate it. I've found out since, it's one of the healthiest things for me.*

> *Nancy: Another assumption I know I made was—I was the only one who wanted healthy foods. When I told my husband I was going to shop for low-fat meal choices, just for me, he said he wanted to try them, too. This was something we had not discussed before.*

I encourage you to let your dream be known by many. They will become attracted to your vision of aspiring to a higher you, and many may want to join you.

One more assumption concerns our BLT's. You know, those invisible bites, licks and tastes? You think a couple of bites won't actually matter, right? In fact, they don't even count for instance, if you eat while you are standing up. This Twinkie won't hurt me, right? Ha ha! Do you want to make a bet? Taking guesses can become a huge place for denial. If someone followed you around for a week, and collected in a baggie, all the unreported and unacknowledged BLTs, what would be in there?

> *Sarah: I know I make assumptions. I think I wrote down everything I ate during the day, but I'm not always mindful of what I eat while the refrigerator door is open, or if I eat right from an ice-cream container.*

> *Susan: The same thing happens to me, while I am cooking. I forget to record those bites.*

> *Nancy: I like nice, neat portions cut from my lasagna or cake pans. If people don't cut a perfect slice across, I'll eat it to even it out, without thinking.*

> *Bert: My job keeps me on the phone all day. I think I have a handle on my hunger, but sometimes I get so absorbed, my little drawer of munchies mysteriously disappears without my knowing what I've done.*

Left unchecked, little assumptions can easily eat away at your accomplishments. However, when you chose awareness and accountability, success is literally, in the palms of your hands.

#4: ALWAYS DO YOUR BEST

Always do your best—knowing your best is going to be different from one instant to the next. Your best will be different when you are well, compared to when you are under the weather. In every situation, do only your best, and you will keep away from negative self-talk, low self-esteem and regret.

Renowned golfer, Dave Duvall, won the championship at the British-Open in England in 2001. (Interestingly enough, he is more able to play his greatest game, now that he lost almost fifty-pounds.) When he was asked how he captured the coveted-cup, he said he was not looking at his score, or Tiger Woods, or the others he was playing against. Instead, Dave took each shot, and simply tried to do his best.

If you always do your best, you respect your body. Your body is a manifestation of God, and if you honor your body, everything changes for you, as you seek your highest good. What changes will you make, if you always do your best?

> *Susan: I will do nothing to abuse my body. I will tell myself my choices of food and drink are for nutrition and for my best health.*

> *Nancy: I will keep exercise as a daily habit, and I will strive to be at peak performance every hour of every day.*

> *Joan: I will choose my rewards as non-food rewards, and I will stay in control, rather than let food control me.*

> *Bert: I will get back on the horse, even if I fall off.*

Always do your best to keep these four agreements. If you always do your best, you will automatically be impeccable with your word; you will not take things personally; and you will not make assumptions. As a consequence, you will see tremendous results in your life and you will experience astonishing effects on the scale. You will reshape your body, mind and spirit. Your life will change, as promised.

Here is a legacy to live by. It speaks to the challenge to always do your best:

People are often unreasonable, illogical, and self-centered
Forgive them anyway.

If you are kind, people may accuse you of selfish, ulterior motives;
Be kind anyway.

If you are successful, you will win some false friends
and some true enemies;
Succeed anyway.

If you are honest and frank, people may cheat you;
Be honest and frank anyway.

What you spend years building, someone could destroy overnight;
Build anyway.

If you find serenity and happiness, they may be jealous;
Be happy anyway.

The good you do today, people will often forget tomorrow;
Do good anyway.

Give the world the best you have, and it may never be enough;
Give the world the best you've got anyway. ⟹

You see, in the final analysis, it is between you and God;
It was never between you and them anyway.

~Engraved on a wall at Mother Teresa's Home for Children
in Calcutta, India~

Did you know you could be a volume eater, and lose weight at the same time? Be sure to read the next chapter to find out about "magical" NEGATIVE calories. That's right. The next exciting section reveals...

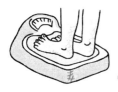 **Chapter Five**

How To Eat MORE — Yet Weigh Less!

BE A "VOLUME" EATER AND LOSE WEIGHT, TOO? Could that be right? Yes, Dear Reader, it is completely true. In fact, I continually eat my husband under the table—yet I remain thin. THIS is the crucial chapter for which you have been waiting. Do read on...

"Fat-and-forty"—they go together. Frightening how your fat creeps on after that age. Somehow, after my fortieth birthday, I got fluffier and fluffier. In fact, I kept packing on more and more pounds, and try as I might, I could not lose weight after that point. Years later, I learned the SECRET. That SECRET helped me lose sixty pounds.

What I discovered is this: men and women, alike, can expect to gain a pound a year after the age of twenty-five. Those who once had an hourglass figure, soon see a shape more like a drooping pear or a round-shaped apple. Nothing changes—(except for more and more weight gain)—unless they do something different to rev up their metabolism.

Here are some shocking statistics:
- Sixty-two percent of our population is overweight.
- More men are overweight than women. (Men lead by four percent—hmmm.)

- After smoking, obesity (thirty pounds or more overweight) is the second-leading cause of avoidable death.
- A study of over one million Americans established a definite connection between obesity and premature death.
- Adult weight gain in women greatly increases their risk for developing cancer of the breast and uterus.
- Adult weight gain in men significantly increases their risk for developing colon and prostate cancer.
- Obese people experience considerably more sickness and disease, as well as forty-four percent greater health-care costs than their slimmer counterparts.

Sadly, most do not know WHY they have gained excess pounds, or HOW to avoid further weight gain. At the time I was battling my own pounds, I didn't know why or how to "rev up" my metabolism, either. The best way I knew to diet was to go on a modified fast. I started each day in earnest, without even eating breakfast. I tried to eat nothing throughout the day until dinner with the family.

Unfortunately, I worked at a mall across from a cookie factory, where the aroma of fresh bakery called constantly to me. Although there were periods when I survived an entire day without giving in to my cravings, there were always the other times when I "broke" the fast. Like the times I saw the bakery girls bagging the goodies from the day before, and reducing them to $1.50 a bag.

What a deal, I thought. I could not let that opportunity go to waste. (*Note the faulty logic. We are often afraid to waste, but the food goes right to our own w-a-i-s-t, and we become the human waste disposal, instead.*) I rationalized I could buy a bargain bag for my family, and eat only one broken cookie during the day, while I was at work.

"Just one cookie—that's all," I promised myself, *"But I most definitely won't eat another."*

"Well—but maybe just one more," a little voice inside of me said...and then it was always one more after that one. Before I knew it, I discretely stuffed down cookie after cookie, in-between customers at my store. More often than not, the sack never came home with me!

No one knew of my good intentions to bring them all a treat, anyway, so there was little harm done, right? As a day like that went by, I continually amazed myself at what a huge eater I actually was. Before long, I started to feel sick and terribly guilty.

Those were usually the nights I ate a light supper when I got home, explaining to everyone: "I'm on a diet." I was crabby, tired, complained of a headache, and went to bed.

What was actually going on?
It's better to start your day with breakfast. Fruit or a fruit smoothie gives an incredible amount of energy, and revs up your metabolism. Your digestive juices go to work on absorbing that energy, while still allowing the food eaten yesterday to digest and leave the body all the sooner.

Throughout your day, it is better to snack on sensible things than to wait and starve. Bring a "survival kit" of finger foods, like veggies and fruits, and a sandwich on wheat or whole grained bread. On an empty stomach, one bite of a cookie will wake up a sleeping monster. White flour and sugar (as found in the cookies) create an adrenalin rush, awakening cravings for more and more. Then comes the crash. It's like an alcoholic's binge. He's fine until he has one drink. Then he craves more and more. After that comes the hangover.

Other times I could fast through the entire day without giving a single thought to the smell of those cookies. I wouldn't realize until I walked out to the parking lot at the end of my day—I was ravenous. So on my way home from work, I would sometimes stop at a fast-food drive-thru, and get something to take home to the family. The ninety-nine cent burgers always seemed like a good deal. *(Once again, note the faulty logic. If I invested a few dollars more, I would have bought better health.)* I'd often get "four burgers to go."

Now, this may have worked, had I put them in the trunk. However, they smelled so yummy, sitting on the seat next to me on the long commute home I would often give in, and take just one. But then, I'd still have a long way to go, and I found I was even hungrier. So I would eat another—and yet another. Subsequently, with only one left, I figured, "I've already blown it—I might as well eat the fourth."

Then to cover up, I would stop at yet another drive-thru, toss away the empty bag, and order four more. When I got home with the burgers, I'd hand them over to the family, and they'd say, *"Aren't you going to eat with us, Mom?"*

"No thanks!" I would say. *"You know I'm on a diet."*

They were always kind enough not to ask why I wasn't losing any weight. But I never lost a pound. In fact, I just gained more.

What was really going on?
Again, it's better to snack on sensible things throughout your day, than to wait and starve. On an empty stomach, one bite of white flour (a hamburger bun), or something fatty (the hamburger patty), or sugary (catsup) will wake up a "Halloween monster." White flour, sugar, and fat all create an adrenalin rush, awakening cravings for more and more. On an empty stomach, logic goes out the window. Then comes the letdown. It's like an alcoholic's splurge. He's okay until he has just a sip. Then he requires another and another. After that come the guilt and self-punishment with more and more.

I was hopeless. I could never lose weight! On the other hand, my daughter, Becky, always took a "pass" on the hamburgers. Yet she ate mounds of food, and stayed skinny and satisfied. Sometimes I would look at her in amazement—eating from her huge, family-sized salad bowl. She piled it high with all kinds of unusual things she brought home. I wondered how she did it. Becky, who was studying to be a nutritionist at the time, always said to me: *"Mom, it's not how MUCH you eat, it's WHAT you eat!"*

I dismissed her comments back then, because I never took much interest in eating fruits and vegetables. I thought she was some kind of a "health nut." Besides, when I was growing up, my family consumed mainly meat, potatoes and gravy. Fruits and veggies were always boring and tasteless to me as a child, so I hardly ever bought them as an adult.

Since then, I have come full circle. I uncovered the SECRET and my daughter was right. What I found is this: certain foods "reverse" calories. The more you eat of them, the more you lose. These foods break down fat, and even counter the effect of fattening foods. They require more calories to digest than they contain. One such example is fresh pineapple. Four ounces contain seventy-six calories. Yet your body uses one hundred calories to digest it. That means twenty-four calories are burned from your own body fat!

There are many such foods that actually take weight from your body. (See them listed in the next chapter.) They force your body to burn its own fat. Because they hasten weight loss, it is more important to eat an enormous amount of these foods than to choose to eat non-fat burning foods with fewer calories. A diet of five to nine cups of fresh or frozen (not canned) fruits and veggies per day, or two-and-a-half to three pounds daily of these fat-blasting foods will create a certain weight loss. It's all of the other foods that are largely responsible for all of your unwanted pounds.

I found I could eat an amazing amount of the foods listed later in the coming chapter, yet I still lost sixty pounds. I am now at my ideal weight, and I have not been this slim since high school. Since that time, I have become a diet enthusiast, and I want to help others. Each week I tell my secrets to hundreds of people who are battling with the same "fat-over-forty" syndrome. They are often astounded at how much I can eat without gaining weight.

If you could change SEVEN BAD CHOICES, all of your weight problems would be solved. Your poor choices often stem from mindless routines, rituals, patterns or customs.

The SEVEN BAD CHOICES SPELL **FAILURE**:

1. **F OODS** with **F**orbidden **F**at
   i.e.: sausage, pork, ham and greasy, battered or fried foods.
2. **A BUNDANCE** of butter and white (not wheat) bread. *They awaken cravings and lead to more.*
3. **I NSISTANCE** on decadent desserts.
   They provide no real nutrition. Find low-calorie substitutes, instead.
4. **L OADS** of creamer, sugar and coffee.
   They slow your weight loss. They retain water.
5. **U SE** of **U**nnecessary salt.
   Contributes to bloating and high blood pressure.
6. **R ITUAL** of **R**equiring **R**ich fats: dressings, cheeses, gravies and sauces. *All of these lead to high cholesterol, high blood pressure and fat.*
7. **E XCUSES** for not **E**xercising; **E**xtinguishing thirst by **E**ating. *Proper exercise and plenty of water will help you to lose weight and keep it off.*

Once your extra weight is lost, the magic foods described later in the next chapter will allow you to live a life as a thin person, yet still have a few of the above fatty foods, without regaining weight. The reason is the fat-demolishing foods do just that—they destroy fat. They bind to other fattening foods, make them less fattening and carry them out of your body before their calories can be stored.

That is why eating ice cream or candy between meals is more fattening than eating them during meals. However, when fibrous foods with minus-calorie value are eaten along with fattening foods, the fibers, which contain pectin, bond to higher-calorie foods. (Think of how pectin is used to solidify jelly or jam.) A large amount of fat and other waste is attached together and carried out of the body. Remember the concept of "beef in a leaf." Wrap beef (a fatty food) in a lettuce leaf (which contains pectin). The pectin bonds to the fat, and leaves the body faster, without doing as much harm. So eat salad all the way through your meal, or to eat an apple along with your dessert.

The magic fat-dissolving foods in the next chapter whisk away excess pounds because they contain fiber. FIBERS are FRIENDS. (CALORIES are CULPRITS.) High fiber foods are automatic weight controllers. Even if you are not on a diet, the simple addition of high fiber foods will tend to normalize your weight, and help you lose pounds and inches if you are too heavy.

High fiber foods act like a "roto-rooter." They sweep up all the poisons in your body. Their soluble fibers enter your blood stream and clear away the cobwebs and the cavern-like build-up of plaque in your veins. If you could see a cross-section of what cholesterol build-up in your veins and intestines looks like, you would be reminded of a spooky cave with stalagmites hanging down and stalactites poking up. Those kinds of formations are the plaque that causes heart disease, high blood pressure, and many other disorders, including cancer.

Without fiber in your diet, the build-up of waste in your colon can become hardened, cling to the walls and fill its many pockets and folds. This results not only in weight gain, but decay and gas, forming slow poisoning of your entire body. It is said John Wayne was found with forty-five pounds of built-up fecal matter in his body when he died. Proper diet could have changed that. (Pardon me, but do you think that explains his famous walk?)

As I look back on my ignorant life of eating all the wrong cuisine, I see my food selections resulted in my own weight gain, and other health problems, as well. For years my doctor warned me:

"Your high blood pressure and frightening cholesterol levels are due to fatty foods in your diet."

"You know I inherited both those problems from my parents," I would always rationalize.

"Never mind that. What are YOU doing these days for exercise?"

"I walk a lot," I'd repeatedly lie.

"If you would step it up a bit, you would see less of your troubles with asthma and arthritis," he explained with each yearly check-up.

"Okay", I'd promise.

"...And start eating more fresh vegetables and fruits."

"Yeah, yeah, OK, Doctor," I'd respectfully reply, while squirming to get out of his office quickly.

All of his warnings fell on my deaf ears. I was unwilling to appreciate his advice. Years later, when I was diagnosed with cancer of my left kidney, I did not even consider there might be a link to the greasy, fried and battered foods I loved and to the vegetables and fruits I was NOT eating. Only now, since I've changed my life around, do I understand—we all have the power to live a healthy life. Our CHOICES create the difference.

Can you defy age? Increase your life span? Protect yourself from cancer, high blood pressure, arthritis, heart disease, diabetes or other health problems and diseases? Avoid "fat-after-forty?" The answer is a resounding—"YES!" Read on, Dear Reader, read on, because prevention is literally in your hands, so long as you can rebuke...

THOSE RASCAL FREE RADICALS

 FREE RADICALS are the ruffians that ravage your body and your health. Numerous problems are caused by what many scientists now refer to as free radicals. Very few individuals, if any, reach their potential maximum life span. They die instead, prematurely, of a wide variety of diseases—the vast majority being free radical diseases.

Regrettably, these rebellious rascals are all over the place. They are in the foods you eat, the water you drink, and the air you breathe. Your body even creates the rousing roughnecks. These riotous rogues consist of a single electron looking for another with which to mate. These fierce aggressors are amazingly productive. Just one rude free radical left unhindered, can cause multiple new ones to emerge. These riffraff, in turn, create countless others.

They beat and bang against your cell walls and create all kinds of chaos, including: allergy, aging, cataracts, heart disease, arthritis, cancer, and countless other conditions, including FAT. Since free radical ruin promotes disease and shortens life, you want to see where these racketeers come from and how to get them OUT of your body as soon as possible. You need to know ways to avoid them. (All the answers are found in the foods in the upcoming chapter.)

Otherwise, over time, these wild hooligans cause chaos in almost any organ or system in your body. Their damage leads to all sorts of degenerative sickness and disease. Free radicals are longevity's most fiendish enemy. They are powerful, microscopic bullets that tear into cell membranes and slash holes into them. The damage these raving rowdies make blasts puncture wounds in a cell's outer wall, letting its inner contents seep out and die. The slippery scoundrels bang into a cell's DNA molecules, wounding and changing them, so they reproduce improperly. If the cell loses its power to reproduce, or replicates abnormally, the process is known as mutation. Mutation can create irregular cells known as cancer.

But cancer is not the only disaster for which free radicals are responsible. Free radical damage is the cause of everything from allergies to heart disease to wrinkles, and a lot more, including FAT. Enough about the ruthless rioters, the remorseless FREE RADICALS. It is time to applaud your ALLIES...

THE AWESOME ANTIOXIDANTS

ANTIOXIDANTS are found in the vitamins and minerals found in the foods in the next chapter. They are your awe-inspiring answer to amazing health. They are like your atomic armed forces. They stand guard, ready to defend your cells against those enemy particles known as the regrettable FREE RADICALS. Antioxidants are the "angels" that lengthen your life span. They create a barrier against heart disease, cancer, and other diseases. They improve your immune system. They contain nutrients that protect against OXIDATION, the process by which free rowdy radicals snatch electrons from healthy cells.

Just as plenty of antioxidants lengthen your life, a lack snatch away your years. The more antioxidants you have in your bloodstream, and defending your cells, the more you can look forward to a longer, happier, healthier life. Before you read about the following POWER foods, which contain these astounding antioxidants, consider the following guidelines to reshape your way to your dreams.

Change SEVEN BAD CHOICES that spell **FAILURE** to SEVEN GOOD CHOICES and your results will spell **SUCCESS**. All your weight problems will be solved. Your old choices, which often stemmed from mindless rituals, patterns or customs, will replace new successful habits on the spot.

SEVEN GOOD CHOICES SPELL **SUCCESS**:

S **UBSTITUTE** **S**pices for **S**alt
U **NDERSTAND** *forbidden foods **U**ndo progress
C **UT** **C**heeses, fats, sauces, dressings and gravies.
C **HOOSE** to discard **C**offee, **C**reamer and sugar.
E **XERCISE** and **E**xtinguish hunger by **E**njoying water.
S **KIP** that Petit Fore.
S **LIP** in more veggies and fruit.

(*Remember the forbidden foods are: pork, ham, sausage, greasy, fried and battered foods.)

...And now...be sure to read and use the knowledge you uncover in the next exciting chapter. Discover rarely known food secrets that could change the length and quality of your life. Learn the...

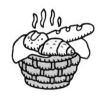

Chapter Six

Foods To Eat More —
Yet Weigh Less!

**THE POWER FOODS-
YOUR GARDEN OF
EDEN**
Start by eating at least five to
nine servings of these foods each
day. You will see a change in
your body, your mind and your
spirit. I promise!

~ALFALFA SPROUTS~

Alfalfa sprouts take up space—in your tummy. They are
great to pile high on a sandwich, or to make as little nests
to surround a salad. They have few calories, no sodium and
they contain an unbeatable source of calcium. Furthermore,
they act as a natural hormone replacement to help control

hot flashes in women. (Because they contain boron, an essential ingredient to bone and joint health, they have many of the same benefits found in artificial hormone replacement, but without the side effects.) Alfalfa sprouts are also excellent for arthritis.

~APPLES~

Did you ever notice when you snack on apples, you feel fuller, longer? Keep them in your car in your "survival kit." They will keep you satisfied, when you are on the road. You won't feel the need to pull into the nearest fast food restaurant to ask for the "super size." Apples are a dense, water-based treat. Their fiber contains pectin, the same ingredient used to thicken jellies and jams. When pectin enters your digestive system, it binds to fat and other "nasties" to form a gel, and out they go! The same gel acts as a double magnet to reduce cholesterol, and high blood pressure. Diabetics can eat apples because the pectin steadies blood sugar levels without a sudden high-low rush.

There's a good reason for the old saying: "an apple a day keeps the doctor away." In truth, an apple a day also keeps the oncologist away. The apple's pectin and fiber crush cancer cells and stop tumors from growing. The skin has an added benefits—it relieves constipation and keeps you regular. It also gives you plenty of awesome antioxidants to keep you looking young, and help keep your joints protected from arthritis.

If you are debating between eating the fruit and drinking the juice, always opt for the fruit. Not only will it fill you up, but it will also provide more fibers to flush away fat and unwanted pounds.

~APRICOTS~

Apricots deserve an "A" because they contain vitamin A, one of the strongest antioxidants known. Vitamin A wards off colds and infections. It also protects your eyes from the reckless free radicals that can stick to artery walls and cause blindness and cataracts.

Apricots will keep you looking young. They contain age-assaulting antioxidants, which reverse the effects of the ravaging free radicals. The mighty antioxidants avenge and avert those rebel ruffians before they can accomplish any recklessness. Apricots halt heart disease. They provide potassium, which frees built-up sodium and clogged arteries. They also help combat cancer. For a dieter, they are a source of quick energy—far more nutritious than any candy bar. The fresh fruit is always best, but dried apricots are quite good, too.

~ARTICHOKES~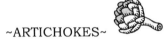

The greatest thing about this vegetable is it takes time and exercise to eat it. (Don't forget—your brain is a laggard, and does not know you have eaten until twenty minutes after the fact, so slow eating is essential to a dieter.) However, artichokes provide tremendous health benefits. The leaves have a lot of fiber to help lower your cholesterol. They help your liver produce more bile, which is helpful for indigestion and stomachache.

For quick cooking of an artichoke (or any vegetable) place it in a cellophane bag, like the kind you find in your produce department, twist the top and cook in your microwave about five to seven minutes, or until tender. Dipping the leaves in butter would be counter-productive to losing weight, but spray-butter and or lemon is perfectly delightful.

~ASPARAGUS~

S-h-h, don't tell! Asparagus is a "skinny secret" eaten by many who are required to weigh-in at a healthy weight in order to keep their jobs. They have found this vegetable acts as a natural diuretic.

Eating asparagus lessens your risk of cancer, heart disease and birth defects because of the folate it contains. Folate cuts harmful acids in your blood. If folate levels drop off, damage can take place in the delicate arteries, which send blood to your heart and brain. Folate stops the growth of cancer-causing substances before they can carry out any damage. Asparagus also contains antioxidants which help sop up those dangerous recurrent free radicals, which when left free rebound wildly through your body, rampaging and rupturing holes in your cells, and doing the types of ruin and mutation that can lead to cancer.

For a tasty twist, boil your asparagus until tender but still crispy. Cut into one-inch strips. Toss with toasted sesame seeds, mixed with balsamic vinegar and a dash of olive oil. Makes a yummy dish to share at any potluck. Serve hot or cold.

~AVOCADOS~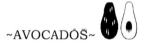

People think avocados are fattening, but half of an avocado a day could actually save your life! The fat contained in an avocado is in fact a good type of fat, and can help make for a healthy heart, skin and joints. The fiber found in this fruit (yes, technically, it is a fruit) will lower your cholesterol, and help prevent stroke, as well as combat cancer. Their potassium helps to lower your blood pressure. Their folate helps your heart, and defends against diabetes.

Try a tasty avocado sandwich on whole-grained bread. To help fill you up, add alfalfa sprouts, cucumber, spinach leaves, tomatoes, garlic powder and mustard. The sandwich is energizing to your body and it uses up lots of digestive energy.

~BANANAS~

Bananas stave off hunger pangs, and leave you fuller longer than most other fruits. I often put a banana in my morning smoothie, and I don't feel a need to eat again until noon. Bananas leave no sugar high, then crashing low.

They contain potassium, which keeps your blood pressure under control and regulates your heartbeat, thus preventing heart attacks, strokes and hardening of your arteries. Potassium thwarts plaque from sticking to your artery walls and blocks harmful cholesterol from oxidizing which causes obstructions to your blood flow. The calcium you get from other foods, needs potassium to create higher bone density, so you build better bones by eating bananas. Bananas also prevent harsh, irritating fluids from causing an upset stomach, or diarrhea. The pectin found in bananas is a soluble fiber, which acts like a sponge in your digestive tract, stimulating the formation of protective mucus.

Need to feel better fast? Reach for a banana—a "happy food" which releases seratonin in your brain. A yummy and sensible way to beat your blues, bananas are crammed with B-6, a vitamin that helps avoid depression. If you have a persistent cough, try a soothing banana.

~BEANS~

"Beans-beans they're good for the heart..." Remember that old childhood chant? Beans are indeed good for your heart, but they have often received a bad rap because they cause gas. A product called "*Beano*" can be used to prevent this discomfort. Many people live with chronic constipation, never recognizing adding beans and other vegetables to their diet could alleviate their problem forever. Their fiber helps keep you "regular," and avoid hemorrhoids, as well as cancer-causing tumors in your colon.

Beans are a good bet for weight loss, too. They satisfy because the fiber fills you up and they have protein to continually replace muscle. They become a complete protein when combined with any grain, such as rice or corn. Since they are high in iron, they are excellent for your blood.

There are many types of beans or legumes from which to choose. They are all good, unless they are prepared with fat or lard. My personal favorite is lentil beans. The best thing about lentils is they don't require pre-soaking before you cook them. They also contain fewer calories than some of the other beans.

~BEETS~

There are many important things to be said about beets. As a dieter, you want to know they can be cooked, prepared and dressed up just like a baked potato, yet they have more fiber and very few calories. All of the beet can be used, even the beet tops, which when chopped small, make a tasty addition to a salad. Eating beets will give you an idea of how long it takes your system to eliminate, so be forewarned because everything that comes out will be a pretty pink.

Beets contain an effective cancer-fighting agent, and the pigment may have anti-tumor forming properties. They also contain the B vitamin, folate, which helps protect against birth defects. Beets have all the nutrients you need for healthy bones. Additionally, their antioxidants help prevent heart disease and high blood pressure.

~BELL PEPPERS~

They are the most nutrient-dense food known. Since your body consists mainly of water, a vegetable like the bell pepper is perfect, because it most closely resembles your body's composition, and will fill you up. Peppers also contain vitamin A, which helps you resist infections and colds. They also soak up and boost the nutrients in other foods you have eaten. Consequently, they improve and enhance every good food choice you make.

Red bell peppers are a "happy" food because they raise your brain levels of serotonin, a chemical that acts as a mood enhancer, and can keep your frame-of-mind sunny and bright. Best of all—bell peppers are rich in silicon, which means beautiful hair, skin, nails and teeth.

~BERRIES~

They're high in fiber, yet they satisfy your sweet cravings. Add fat-free whipped topping, and they taste like a sinful dessert. These are nature's own candies, but you can eat plenty of them without guilt, because your body hardly absorbs the calories. Berries are an "age-buster" food. Since they are high in antioxidants, they combat free radicals all night long, and their anti-aging powers make your skin beautiful and smooth. Your wrinkles just seem to fade and you look years younger.

What makes berries so special? They contain a compound, a sort of elixir, which prevents organic changes that can lead to cancer. It is a powerful antioxidant, which can reduce the damage caused by free radicals, the harmful oxygen molecules that can knock holes in healthy cells and jolt the beginning of the harmful cancer process. The nutrient actually detoxifies carcinogens. Berries are also very high in vitamin C, which is one of the most powerful antioxidants. Getting a lot of vitamin C may lower your peril of heart disease and infections. Vitamin C seems particularly important in preventing cataracts, which are caused by the oxidation of the protein that forms the lenses of your eyes.

Berries also relieve constipation. They contain large amounts of insoluble fiber, which is incredibly absorbent. Their fiber draws large amounts of water into the intestine, which makes for better elimination. Berries also stop bile acid (a chemical your body uses for digestion) from being changed into a more perilous, potentially cancer-causing form of acid.

For a great start in your morning, blend frozen strawberries or blueberries into your smoothies. (Soymilk and tofu give a smooth and healthy base.)

~BREAD~ (whole wheat or whole grained—NOT white bread)

Don't be afraid to eat bread—whole wheat bread, or whole grained bread, that is. It reduces your appetite, makes you feel fuller longer, and is the best steady fuel. Keep the wheat choice in mind when it comes to picking tortillas, pasta, and buns, too. That's because wheat (not white) contains lots of fiber. White breads have more sugar and processing, and in effect create cravings, which are hard to quiet. Be sure the ingredients contain whole wheat, or whole grain because a lot of breads labeled "wheat bread" are only white bread with caramel coloring.

Wheat also contains vitamin E, an important vitamin in fighting those rascally free radicals. Vitamin E plays an important part in lowering your cholesterol, preventing it from sticking to the walls of your arteries. Wheat also contains protein, something you'll want to be sure to have a certain amount of in order to hang onto your muscle mass as you continue to lose or maintain your weight.

Wheat is a whole grain high in fiber and low in fat. That means it's ideal for the dieter. Populations consuming large amounts of whole grains have lower rates of breast, colon and prostate cancers, as well as diabetes.

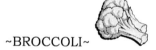

~BROCCOLI~

Broccoli is America's most-favored veggie, cooked or raw. Even though it wasn't a favorite of a former president of the United States, it should be one of your own best liked because it is the number one cancer-fighting vegetable. Those little flowers are exceptionally powerful in closing down cancers of the colon, prostate and breast. The antioxidants sweep up cancer-causing elements prior to their doing any harm. The antioxidant combinations found in broccoli are extremely effective in confronting breast cancer. They lower levels of damaging estrogens that can encourage tumor development in hormone-sensitive cells, like breast cells. The agents boost the creation of cancer-blocking enzymes.

Broccoli is also chocked-full of more common compounds like beta-carotene to lower rates of heart attack and cataracts. Because it contains calcium, it is also a great way to combat osteoporosis. It has plenty of calcium, to build better bones. Broccoli also contains Folate, one of the B vitamins, which helps to combat Alzheimer's disease, depression and birth defects. (Women, especially those who take birth control pills, are often low in this vital nutrient.) Be on the lookout for broccoli sprouts, too. They contain many times more vitamins and antioxidants.

Many people experience discomfort and gas when first eating too much of this vegetable, which incidentally, also protects against hemorrhoids and diabetes. It would be best to keep an open mind, introduce quantities gradually, and ask your pharmacist to recommend an over-the-counter relief.

~CABBAGE~

Want a superb weight loss? Try making several big pots of homemade cabbage soup, along with a whole lot of your other favorite fresh veggies and spices. Use this healthy, hearty soup as an entire meal or as a snack to fill you up, and watch your pounds disappear quickly. (You might see as much as five pounds vanish in a week).

Cabbage protects against colon, breast and prostate cancers. The invaluable compounds it contains sweep up hurtful hormones, as well as block harmful cells from growing by stepping up the creation of tumor-preventing enzymes in your body. Study shows toxins are swept out of your body before they have a chance to damage the delicate cells lining the intestinal wall.

Although eating vegetables raw is always preferred, with cabbage, it doesn't matter how long you cook it. For the best nutrients, try bok choy or savoy. Eating cabbage may increase your life span. It has also been known to heal ulcers and ease constipation.

~CANTALOUPE~

Cantaloupe, like asparagus, is another "secret" food known by many weight loss support group staff members who eat it before their monthly weigh-in. That is because it is a natural diuretic. The soluble fiber works lots of other magic, too, including saving your eyesight, combating cancer, controlling blood pressure and lowering cholesterol. Nutritionists even suggest cantaloupe for diabetics because of its heart-friendly effects. Watermelon is a similar fruit with lots of water and fiber to fill you up, yet low in calories.

~CARROTS~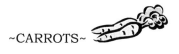

Many of us heard as children eating carrots helps your eyesight. Well, it's true, and as you age, that fact becomes more and more important, since you may experience loss of vision or night blindness. Carrots contain beta-carotene, a powerful cancer-fighting agent, as well as a compound that converts into vitamin A and helps improve vision.

Get your kids to eat more veggies now. If they say "Yuck!" here's a trick: You all know how everyone loves pasta—it's your way to a man's and a kid's heart. Just add carrots to spaghetti sauce for a natural sweetener. No one will know. Then, the next time, start slipping other veggies into the sauce, too.

While most vegetables are more nutritious raw than cooked, carrots benefit from a little cooking, as the fibers are then more easily absorbed. Cooked carrots also act as a great choice for older persons who have trouble chewing or who experience gas from other vegetables.

Carrots are tasty because they contain some sugar, but as a diet food, they are superior. The amounts of fiber they contain restore regularity and fend off heart disease, as well as lung and breast cancer. They scarf-up the scavenging free radicals before they can do any harm. Carrots make a great finger food. Keep some on hand to ward off a "snack attack."

~CAULIFLOWER~

Just like broccoli, cauliflower is one of the best cancer fighting foods. It is a cruciferous vegetable that fights tumors. It is especially protective against breast and prostate cancers. Cauliflower builds strong bones to avoid fractures and osteoporosis. It is also extremely valuable in keeping the immune system strong. That's because it is packed with lots of vitamin C and folate. It's often recommended for people who are anemic, and helps to banish bruises. The newly introduced "brocco-flower" has even more vitamins than either cauliflower or broccoli.

~CEREAL~

Pick a high-fiber cereal, instead of the old *"Fruit Loops"* choice. Some cereals have eight grams or more per serving. My personal favorite is *"Kashi Just Friends."* It takes a long time to digest and keeps me fuller longer, helping to stave off the munchies. It's even good as an evening snack, along with a diet pudding, and fat-free topping. Add a maraschino cherry and it becomes something like a decadent dessert. All that fiber can act like a sponge in your digestive tract and prevent other calories from being absorbed.

~CHICKEN~

Don't eat the skin and you'll have a complete protein—a far healthier choice than meats like beef or pork that slow you down and make you sluggish and sleepy. Chicken is also an excellent source of iron, niacin and zinc, the other B vitamins, which, if you lack them, you'll find yourself coming down with every germ, as well as low energy, slow memory, and mood swings.

As with any meat or fish, be sure to watch portion control, use as condiments, rather than as the main event. It is best to combine your meals with plenty of fresh fruits, vegetables and grains. A well-balanced diet containing plenty of antioxidants containing vitamins A, C and E will help absorb and digest the fat from the chicken.

There has been increased concern when you eat chicken, you also take in the same growth-stimulating hormones, antibiotics, and toxins the bird did. Therefore, it is best to know the highest source for protein would be beans or soybeans.

~CHILI PEPPERS~

Kick your salt habit by substituting chili peppers. Rev up your spice and you rev up your metabolism. According to experts, the hotter the pepper, the better it is for your health and your weight loss. In fact, peppers speed up your whole digestive process. They stimulate protective digestive juices to flow, and get your stomach muscles moving to prevent poor digestion and ulcers in your intestinal tract.

They also lower your cholesterol and triglyceride levels, and act as an anti-aging armory against free radicals that can cause damage and create heart disease, stroke, arthritis and a weakened immune system. Chili peppers are red-hot in vitamins A and C. Peppers will help thin your blood to protect against heart attack. Their many healing powers include a natural decongestant, helping to thin mucus due to coughs and colds. Chili peppers can also soothe and numb a sore throat.

~CORN~

Corn is low in calories and high in fiber and packed with water, so it will fill you up and give you energy. Corn on the cob is hard to eat quickly, so you are not likely to eat too much. If you are of the opinion corn is fattening, it might be because you've always eaten it with butter and salt. Try one of the spray butters instead (with zero sodium, calories and fat), and if you still need the salt, try a salt substitute. Eat corn with beans for a complete protein. White corn is best because it has more fibers. Eating corn helps fight high blood cholesterol and heart disease.

~CRANBERRIES~

If you are prone to urinary infections, have cranberry juice frequently, and it will be a natural way to fight back bacteria from being able to stick to the walls of your urinary tract. Whole cranberries also have anti-cancer powers, and prevent heart disease, ulcers and gum disease. Their pigment contains nonstick flavonoids, which prevent dangerous forms of bacteria from clumping together.

~FIGS~

Now, here's the perfect food for a diet. Figs prevent overeating because they make you feel fuller longer. Figs mean fiber. Bite into those tiny seeds and you know you have experienced something healthy—like eating a strawberry inside out. They will keep you satisfied, and you'll eat less of other fattening foods. They're a great source of energy, and calcium, too. Plus, they're a natural laxative, and a beneficial treat for diabetics because all that fiber lowers their glucose levels.

~FISH~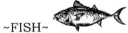

If you want to get <u>thin</u>, eat things that <u>swim</u>. There are far greater benefits in fish than experts first imagined. Not only does fish have the least amount of calories compared to chicken or beef, but it also fills you up longer because of its high water content. Several meals of fish per week help keep your heart healthy, your arteries open, and reduce your chance of heart attacks. The beneficial oils in fish reduce stiff joints caused by arthritis. Their healthy omega 3 oils thin your blood, reduce blood pressure and lower cholesterol. Fish in your diet can reduce your chance of cancer and stroke, as well. Ask any Eskimos—they'll know.

As with any meat or fish, be sure to watch portion control. It is best to combine your meals with plenty of fresh fruits and vegetables. A well-balanced diet containing plenty of antioxidants containing vitamins A, C and E will help absorb and digest the fat from the fish.

A word of caution: Controversy continues regarding many fish found to be swimming in toxins. Those same harmful chemicals can be passed on to humans. The best source of protein would still be soybeans.

~GARLIC~

Many people love garlic for the taste. You will love it even more when you discover garlic combats many diseases. Garlic's health-giving properties are unmatched by any other single food. Give it to someone who has persistent bronchitis, as it has been known to kill germs and bacteria. Garlic is a great natural antibiotic, much like penicillin. It works well as an expectorant and a decongestant, and will stimulate your immune system. You will find you have less colds and infection if you eat plenty of garlic.

Garlic also contains cancer-preventive agents. Studies show garlic can help block cancer in several ways: by preventing cell changes that lead to cancer, by stopping tumors from growing, and by killing the harmful cells outright. The substance found in garlic acts as a throttle to the growth of cancer cells by interfering with their ability to divide and multiply. It basically chokes cancer cells until their numbers are reduced and they start dying. It is one of the most potent tumor suppressors known. Combining three to six cloves of garlic a day with your food could reduce your risk of many cancers.

Garlic stops blood clots. The herb promotes smooth blood flow by preventing platelets from sticking together, thereby reducing your risk of heart attacks and strokes. It can actually help reverse some of the effects. It also assists in managing cholesterol.

Eat it fresh or powdered (fresh is always best), as a tasty addition to stir-fries, salads, or pasta—or roast it and spread it on bread. Put it in your microwave for just a few seconds to cut the strong taste. If you're worried people will stay away from you because you smell of garlic, add lemon and parsley for even more added health.

~GRAPEFRUIT~

Grapefruit contains a host of age-busting antioxidants. The chemical make-up dissolves fat and cholesterol. The pectin it produces acts as a "roto-rooter", cleaning your pipes to fight against hardening of your arteries. Can' t sleep at night? Try the juice—it's capable of promoting sound slumber. Grapefruit also inhibits constipation. If your doctor says you have too much bad cholesterol, grapefruit will help to restore your good to bad cholesterol ratio.

~GRAPES and WINE made with grape skins~

Grapes are an easy finger-food for a dieter. Take them anywhere and they will keep you satisfied, and make a welcome addition to any potluck. Because they are dense with water and nutrients, they make a better choice than raisins, which contain more calories and less volume. Try freezing grapes for a refreshing snack. They'll last longer and you'll eat less.

The real secret in grapes is found in their skins. Grape skins hold plant estrogen and other antioxidants, which perform like superstars. The compounds found in grapes help to block cholesterol from building up in your artery walls. They also help to ward off the threat of cancer, age-related loss of vision, and kidney stones. The same can be said of red wine, because it is made with grape skins during the fermenting process. Many doctors agree drinking wine in moderation can reduce your risk of heart attack, heart disease and stroke.

~KALE~

You will never leave it on your plate again as just a pretty decoration—not when you discover kale rated highest in amounts of antioxidants over any other vegetable. Kale can absorb more of those damaging free radicals and sweep them (along with fat) right out of your body.

Kale contains one of the best plant sources of easily absorbed calcium and vitamin K. That means kale helps prevent osteoporosis and risk of bone fracture. Eating kale protects your eyes from cataracts and macular degeneration. Here's more good news: Kale prevents cancer from forming. Eat it fresh or cooked, but be sure to never pass it up—at your produce department or on your plate.

~KIWI~

Kiwis make a pretty addition to any salad, and will slice easily with a heavy-duty egg slicer. They're free of fat and sodium. They are ideal for someone with elevated blood pressure because their tiny seeds contain high fiber. An added benefit: kiwis help chase away constipation.

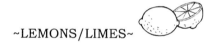

~LEMONS/LIMES~

Did you ever notice many Oriental people cook with lemons and limes? Did you ever notice those same people are almost all exceptionally slim, healthy and have beautiful skin? Hmmmm. Well, for one thing, citrus fruits contain an acid that acts as a catalyst to proteins and causes more efficient burning of calories. Remember the old "Stewardess diet?" It was very similar in that it combined a citrus and a protein, such as lemon and chicken, or orange and turkey, grapefruit and egg, or tomato and fish. Add lemon or lime to anything, and it will become a fat-burner.

These citrus fruits contain plenty of age-busting antioxidants, as well. Your skin will take on a healthier glow, if you eat lemons. Add the "zest" or peeling because it contains a chemical that can prevent skin cancer. Lemons and limes also contain vitamin C which helps stop cholesterol build-up in your veins.

~LETTUCE~

Lettuce is packed with carotene and vitamin C. The best picks are the dark green leafy types. Kale has the most calcium of all. Romaine and red leaf are good bets, too. Iceberg lettuce is often the least expensive, however, it has nowhere near the same nutrients. Wrap anything in lettuce, and it will bind to the pectin found in this vegetable, like a jelly or jam bonds, and leave your body more efficiently. (Remember the concept of beef in a leaf? See the previous chapter.) If you're having a restless night, grab a bunch of lettuce—it's a remedy for restless sleep.

~MANGOES~

Add mango chunks to your morning smoothie—you won't be hungry until noon. Mangoes are excellent for digestion and extremely satisfying. They are chock-full of Vitamin C and other antioxidants that stave off cancer and memory loss. Like citrus fruits, mangoes contain an enzyme that breaks down protein. Use them in a marinade to tenderize meats and avoid cancer. Women find mangoes are great for hot flashes because they decrease body heat. The fruit is a natural deodorant—-able to counteract body odors.

~ONIONS~

Discovering the benefits found in onions will cause you tears of joy. Onions are nutritional powerhouses. They contain amazing antioxidants, including sulfur, a forceful tumor suppressor. These extraordinary vegetables prevent just about every type of cancer.

If your doctor has told you to worry about your cholesterol levels, a cupful of onions a day could improve those numbers, and lower your triglycerides. Onions help cleanse your blood by releasing helpful sulfur compounds that sweep up those reproachful free radicals, preventing them from sticking to your artery walls. They help block clogging of your arteries. One more reason to start eating more onions is they can stop infections and destroy germs, and can even counteract salmonella on the meat you grill.

Are you plagued with allergies or asthma? Try onions and see if they don't decrease your allergic reactions. Onions assist your respiratory system by loosening phlegm. They are also excellent for your liver. Worried about onion breath? Just eat more parsley, and it will do even more for your health! So go ahead, and have an onion on everything.

~ORANGES~

Oranges are straight from "the Garden of Eden." They are the sweetest fruit of all, and nature's own candy. Quick energy is what they provide. But, more importantly, their healthful compounds also help reduce your risk of a number of cancers. Don't hesitate to eat the fluffy white rind, and the seeds, as well. They are jam-packed not only with vitamins, but they also contain other powerful chemicals that deactivate cancer-causing carcinogens.

Oranges are best known for vitamin C, which will controls those harmful, riotous free radicals, but oranges also provide the immune-boosting power of fighting colds. Eating orange lowers blood cholesterol and fights arterial plaque. So, have an orange a day and help insure your health.

What about drinking the juice, instead? If you're trying to lose weight, it's better to fill up on the fresh fruit and the healthful fiber it provides. The juice has more calories, and, besides, any processing removes most of the nutrients.

~PEACHES~

Many older people who complain of gas from fruits and vegetables will be glad to try peaches. They are easy to digest, which is true from babyhood to old age. The large amount of water and high fiber found in peaches makes them helpful in keeping "regular." Try to eat them in season, when they are packed with vitamins.

~PEAS~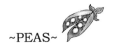

Kids and adults, alike, are naturally drawn to those cute, little green pods. A perfect finger food, the shiny peas inside are packed with healthy vitamins. If your doctor has told you to watch your triglyceride and cholesterol levels, then peas will be a "natural" to add to your diet. They have a cholesterol-lowering soluble fiber. This type of fiber also helps control blood sugar, something diabetics want to know. Inside your intestine, the fiber in peas binds with bile, a digestive fluid produced by your liver, which traps and sends toxins out of your body. Since bile is high in cholesterol, removing it from your body will automatically bring cholesterol levels down. As a result, peas are valuable in keeping hearts strong. Their carotene and vitamin C also promote them as effective little green cancer traps. Peas prevent other diseases, as well, including the common cold.

~PINEAPPLE~

An exceptional diet food, fresh pineapple is loaded with the mineral manganese, which is vital for bone development. Your bones need this mineral to make collagen, a resilient fibrous protein that attaches your connective tissues like bone, skin and cartilage. People missing manganese in their diet can develop osteoporosis.

Pineapple helps ease indigestion, a tip particularly helpful for elderly people who are often limited in the few fruits and veggies they can eat. Certain ingredients in pineapples help the enzymes that breakdown proteins and carbohydrates to aid absorption while soothing your stomach. (If you overindulge, fresh pineapple can decrease your discomfort.)

This tangy tropical fruit has lots of vitamin C, a powerful antioxidant, which will thwart those pesky free radicals that contribute to the development of cancer and heart disease. Vitamin C reduces the levels of histamine, which cause cold symptoms, such as runny noses and watery eyes.

~POPCORN~

When it comes to going on a diet, the most important thing is finding satisfying snacks. Popcorn provides a lot of fiber and hence you feel fuller—longer. Buy popcorn kernels in bulk, without extra seasonings or butter added first. Pop your popcorn dry in a microwave popper or a brown paper bag. Or use an air-popper. Use non-fat spray butter if you are missing flavor. Instead of salt, use non-sodium substitutes or spices. You will avoid fat and calories, and see great results in weight loss from the extra fiber.

Don't be tempted to buy popcorn at the movies. It is popped in coconut oil, the most deadly fat. Instead, bring your own popcorn in an unobtrusive shopping bag. I have done this countless times, and no one has ever stopped me. If they do, I'm ready with an answer. I'll simply say: *"I'm allergic to **YOUR** popcorn. It makes me break out—in **FAT**!"*

~POTATOES~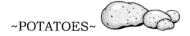

Looking for an excellent food for rapid weight loss? Try potatoes. They are extremely filling, and exceptionally nutritious. What then is the reason many people think of a potato as fattening? It is because of what they add to that "tuber"—things like butter, sour cream and cheese. Try some non-fat spray butter instead, and then add broccoli, onions, maybe some mushrooms and salsa, and you'll have a complete low-calorie, low-fat meal—one that will hold you longer than most other choices.

To get the most out of the potatoes' cancer-combating capabilities, you want to eat the skin. It helps soak up carcinogens from diverse things you may have eaten, especially from grilled, smoked or canned foods. Eating the potato with the skin will also help lower your cholesterol and protect against strokes and heart disease.

The starchy vegetable is not only a great source of fiber but also potassium. Some people are even able to stop taking high blood pressure medication by eating potatoes. In addition to everything else, diabetics will love to know potatoes can keep excess sugar out of their bloodstream. Because potatoes are complex carbohydrates, they must be broken down gradually into simple sugars before entering your bloodstream. As a result, blood sugar levels remain fixed, which is a large factor in regulating diabetes.

Note: Bruises and eyes should be removed from potatoes before cooking, as they may contain harmful compounds.

~PRUNES~

Prunes can boast of more than twice the amount of antioxidants found in any other food. Have a daily dose of seven prunes, and you will greatly reduce your likelihood of aging, wrinkling and forgetfulness.

Prunes are fiber powerhouses. Add prunes to your daily diet and you'll be a "regular" type of guy (or gal). Prunes bring about regularity through their insoluble fiber, which is the secret to avoiding constipation. Your body does not absorb insoluble fiber—it stays in your digestive tract. Since this kind of fiber is amazingly absorbent, it sops up massive quantities of fluid. Insoluble fiber helps reduce your bad cholesterol and with it your danger of heart disease.

Prunes have a natural sugar called sorbitol, which soaks up water. (Most fruits show modest quantities of sorbitol, but prunes have the most, which makes clear why they are such an enormous bulking feature.) Prunes likewise contain plenty of potassium, a mineral vital for keeping blood pressure low.

~RICE (brown or wild, not white)~

Rice can be your starting point to dramatic weight loss. The most beneficial is brown rice, which contains rich amounts of fiber. The external covering of brown rice is enveloped in a vitamin-laden outer-skin. This jacket is the section of the grain highest in fiber. (White rice is processed, and has removed the best part.) It contains a substance similar to cholesterol-lowering prescriptions. In blending with a low-fat diet, brown rice is one of the greatest foods you can feast on and cut your cholesterol at the same time.

The fiber in brown rice is the insoluble kind that acts the same as a sponge mop in your intestine, soaking up enormous amounts of water. As the fibers collect water, they get hold of any destructive substances, thus giving those relentless free radicals a smaller amount of time to wreak havoc on cells in your intestinal walls. All of this can help put a stop to your threat of cancer. The fiber in brown rice also attaches itself to estrogen right in the intestine, so there are a smaller amount of harmful hormones moving about in the bloodstream. This is critical since high amounts of estrogen have been made known to step up abnormal reorganization in breast cells and that can lead to cancer.

Rice is an excellent source of phosphorus and protein. It reduces kidney ailments and high blood pressure.

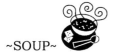

~SOUP~

There is magic in soup. It is your greatest "skinny secret" of all. To get your best results, it should be homemade with fresh ingredients. Canned and dried soups have too much sodium and processing to have the same results. As a weight support group leader, I recommend new members make a pot of delicious homemade vegetable soup. The more they eat, the more they lose. The average first-week weight loss is often five pounds or more. The reason is they are able to fill up on the soup, and if they throw in a head of cabbage, it acts as a natural diuretic and laxative. Hot soup has to be eaten slowly, so it tends to be more filling, since it takes your brain about twenty minutes to register your stomach has been fed. (Find Soup Recipe in Chapter 9.)

~SOYBEANS~

Soy to the World! Soy is healthful to both men and women. Soy is rich in natural compounds dubbed as phytoestrogens, which your body changes into hormone-like materials that perform like a weak form of estrogen. Soy foods include a compound, which restrains the development of tumors by stopping blood vessels from developing in the surrounding area. Soy foods provide your most powerful cancer protection available. In fact, soy can prevent just about every type of cancer. Even more amazing, soy foods can actually help coax cancer cells to return to normal.

In pre-menopausal women, soybeans can help lessen chances of breast cancer. In later life, women find soybeans reduce hot flashes, mood swings and "PMS." However, one of the most vital problems facing women is the possibility of their bones fracturing after menopause. Soy foods can make the difference. Phytoestrogens found in soy are a weaker plant form of female estrogen. These hormone-like materials take an active part in helping bones retain calcium, even when they are no longer generating estrogen.

Men benefit from soy, too. By using soy products in the diet, they are less likely to develop prostate cancer. Soy helps curb dangerous effects of the male hormone, testosterone, which is thought to fuel growth of cancerous cells in the prostate gland. Soy hampers the effects and closes off the fuel that stimulates the cancer to generate.

The benefits of soy are endless. Soy is high in protein and calcium, potassium and iron. Soy products are full of compounds that aid in controlling blood pressure, cut cholesterol, lower triglycerides, regulate blood sugar, ease constipation, and even eliminate or dissolve gallstones.

Soy is the only plant food that is a total protein. There are many appealing soybean products at health food and grocery stores these days, it is quite simple to discover a way to fit soy into your diet. There is tofu, made from soy curd, soy burgers, soy crumbles, soy hot dogs, soy cheese, soymilk, soy nuts, and the fresh green soybeans known as edamame, which are found in the soy pods or pre-shucked.

I start my day with a soy smoothie, with soy milk, silken tofu, and any kind of fruit I have around, like a banana, and some age-defying blueberries or strawberries. Lunch could be a soy burger, piled high with tomato, lettuce, or spinach and onion on a wheat bread spread with lots of mustard, (not mayo, unless it is low-fat or no-fat.). Dinner is often a stir-fry with plenty of veggies, including soybeans, and tofu. Soybeans and soy can also be included in soups and casseroles. Add soy to your world.

~SPINACH~

Spinach is a great food for weight-loss because it has the ability to rev up your metabolism. Eat it cooked or raw, and it will decrease cholesterol. It also has a natural laxative effect. Use the flexible leaves to layer any veggie wrap or sandwich, and it won't fall apart.

Spinach is chock full of vitamins and contains antioxidants that protect your eyes from cataracts by protecting your eyes from light damage and supporting the blood vessels to your retinas. The dark green veggie also guards against cancer, especially colon, stomach, lung and breast cancer.

~SWEET POTATOES~

You can build a meal around sweet potatoes and not fret about gaining weight. Their high fiber not only fills you up, but helps control your weight. All that fiber also helps lower your blood pressure and keep your arteries flowing smoothly. Sweet potatoes are also a great food for someone with diabetes, because they help regulate blood sugar.

Because sweet potatoes are a first-rate source of vitamins and additional antioxidants, they are can help cut your possibility of lung and other types of cancer. They contain vitamin E, which is hard to find in other foods. Vitamin E stops free radicals before they cause cancer, heart disease, asthma and arthritis. The bright orange pigment of the sweet potato is loaded with beta-carotene, which disables damaging molecules before they cause damage in certain parts of your eyes. As a result, sweet potatoes could save your eyes from macular degeneration and cataracts.

These bright and tasty "tubers" do magnificent things to boost a bright and sunny disposition. They contain B6, a vitamin that balances chemicals in your brain to release seratonin, a natural mood enhancer. Sweet potatoes also hold ingredients to help stave off osteoporosis.

~TOFU~

Tofu is really soybean curd, so it provides many of the same benefits as soy. That means less hot flashes, mood swings and PMS! Japanese women eat tofu and soy regularly, yet they have no such problems. It is interesting to note they are also slim. Hmmmm.

Tofu also has impressive amounts of calcium and iron. It helps regulate blood sugar, insulin levels and bowel function. Numerous studies have shown tofu helps prevent cancer, especially stomach cancer. Use it in place of meat in your diet, and gain healthful results as you lose weight quickly. Tofu is extremely versatile. It takes on the taste of chicken, fish or beef. Spice it up and throw it in an omelet, stir-fry or sandwich. Keep an open mind, and you may find you like tofu more than you know. It is filling, but what you will like best is what it does for your waistline and your health.

~TOMATOES~

They're loaded with fiber, help you to drop excess pounds and look ever so healthy, radiant and young. In fact, the likelihood of dying of cancer is least among people who eat tomatoes on a daily basis. If you do, you drastically shrink your chances of lung cancer. Men will want to know routinely eating tomatoes offers them a powerful safeguard from prostate cancer. That is because tomatoes contain lycopene, an antioxidant that gives tomatoes their brilliant color. Lycopene, found in only a few plants, has even been known to reverse prostate cancer.

The red pigment in tomatoes also contains anti-aging antioxidants, which offset those rollicking free radicals before they can do any destruction in injuring cell walls. Tomatoes contain plenty of vitamin C to defend against cataracts, heart disease, and depression. They also contain vitamin A to help boost up your resistance to germs.

Use tomatoes as a snack, sauce, or main dish. In a soup or casserole their healthful compounds stand up well to heat. Try the sun-dried variety, or cherry tomatoes, which make a wonderful "squish" in your mouth. In fact, those tiny cherry or grape tomatoes make a convenient finger food, and travel well in your "diet survival kit," if you are a commuter.

~TURNIPS~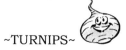

Dieters find a wonderful surprise in turnips. They fill you up as well as potatoes do, but with far less calories. Throw one in a cellophane bag and put it into your microwave for 10 minutes or until soft. Add salsa, spices, spray butter, and whatever else you would to a baked potato, and you will get the same satisfaction, but lose weight all the faster.

Turnips have an incredible amount of potassium. From the cabbage family, turnips hinder tumor formation. They also hold marvelous amounts of vitamins A and C, and contain calcium, iron and protein, as well.

~YOGURT~

Yogurt is a great source of calcium. It's also nature's antibiotic to prevent yeast infections. The helpful bacteria in yogurt are known to strengthen your immune system and to keep ulcer-causing bacteria under control. Not all yogurts are created equal, however. Always check the amount of calories, even if the label says "low" or "no fat".

Feast on the foods just described in this chapter, and you will melt away excess pounds. They are packed with fiber and nutrients. They keep you satisfied, and help you find your ideal weight

Do you remember it takes just twenty-one days to form a new habit? Learn and apply the habits of successful people, because in the next chapter you will find...

The following chapter is an adapted transcript from a seminar led by the author.

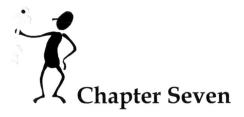

Chapter Seven

The Seven Keys
To A <u>SLIMMER</u> You!

Why is it some people can stay successfully slim? Why is it others can't seem to release weight at all? What are the patterns of slim people? What do they do? You will uncover the answers in this chapter.

Here are the SEVEN KEYS TO A **SLIMMER** new you:

- **S** ee hope.
- **L** ist priorities
- **I** magine yourself slim.
- **M** astermind with others.
- **M** ake time for you.
- **E** xpand your mind.
- **R** espond to your weight.

 KEY #1: **S**ee hope. **S**limmer

See hope of becoming slim. Be convinced you are a successful person. Look at your other successes in all the other areas of your life. Know that you will be successful in managing your weight, as well. If you see hope, you will always look at the glass as half-full, never half-empty. Love and accept yourself from the very start of your journey. Never look in the mirror and say, "I have fat cheeks," or "Gee, I have big thighs!" Consider yourself as a work in progress. Say to yourself, "I'm getting slimmer and slimmer every day." You are victorious simply by deciding to move forward, and saying: "I can do it!" Congratulate yourself on your healthy decision because the best is yet to come.

> *Lon: I see hope because I'm going toward health that's going to make me be the "best me" I can be. Along with releasing the weight, I aspire to be the "best me" I can be on every level, especially in my job, and my relationships with my wife and kids.*

> *Sharon: I feel like a winner, even though I have a lot further to go. I've already let go of thirty pounds, and I've dropped several dress sizes. I feel much better. My doctor is proud of me, and I'm proud of myself.*

> *Susan: I only see good things ahead. I've gotten my whole family to think of making healthy choices, right along with me, and that is a major thing.*

Every single one of you will look better, and feel better— plus you will all live long, happy, healthy lives together. One way we can live a life like that is to have heroes.

One of my greatest heroes through the years, for health, humor, and happiness is Art Linkletter. I try to emulate his wholesome, upbeat spirit and laughter. Do you remember, as I do, laughing until your sides ached at his ***Kids Say the Darndest Things TV Show?*** Laughing, itself, is a great exercise. One hundred good belly laughs a day, over a week, will result in one more pound of weight loss. So, laugh your pounds away!

People who say, "I can't do it!" are the negative people who always see the glass as half-empty. They assume they are going to lose out on life, or they will have to give up something if they change. But you don't have to give up anything. What would you tell those who are afraid they will lose out?

> *Janet: I would tell them to work on their sense of humor. I would also tell those people they could find alternatives for the things they crave. Like, I love Haagen-Dazs ice cream, but I've found a healthier ice-cream choice, and I don't feel deprived at all. I even treat myself once a week to a hot-fudge sundae, and then I make up for it by trading it off, on another day.*

> *Morey: I used to be the sedentary, negative one in our marriage. Now, my wife has given me a new mind-set. She has helped me lose twenty-eight pounds, recently, by encouraging me and reminding me—food is not the reward—the real reward is being able to take control of my life. Now, we both have a winning situation, as I am more able to participate and enjoy activities along with my family.*

By replacing some of our old patterns with healthier choices we can see results that are lifesaving. It is about knowing what is important, which bring us to our next key...

 KEY #2: **L**ist priorities. s**L**immer

List your priorities each day. Put yourself first. Decide to tackle first what is most important, and that is YOU. Put your goals first. How often do we neglect to do this? At the end of each day, check off each item listed with a <u>V</u> for Victory. Plan your day. Harvey Mackay says it all in **Pushing the Envelope**: *"People don't plan to fail, they fail to plan."*

Too often we become mesmerized in other day-to-day things. One thing that gets in the way of our priorities is TV. Statistics concerning the amount of television watching we do is staggering. Stephen R. Covey in his book, **The Seven Habits of Highly Effective People**, reports the average person in his lifetime will watch sixteen years of television. The typical family has the television on for eight to eight-

and-a-half hours a day. That's equivalent to a full-time job. Your "little black box" can be addicting, like food. It contributes to a sedentary life-style, and can get in your way of your goal toward weight loss. So, in putting yourself first, you have a multitude of things you could put foremost, instead, rather than getting lured into one more half-hour show. For that reason, put first, the things that would move you closer to what you really want.

So...do you have a plan each day for exercise? Do you make a date with yourself, just as you would plan a date with someone else? Do you plan to leave the house each day with a survival kit packed with healthy finger foods like grapes, cherry tomatoes, apples and things that will keep you satisfied while you are on the road, so you won't be tempted to pull over to the nearest fast food restaurant and ask for the super-size? Do you plan a way to get in your five to nine daily servings of fruits and veggies? Do you plan a list of the healthy foods you need when you go to the grocery store? Do you arrive hungry at a party? Do you have a plan for risky restaurants, risky people, or risky events? Failure to plan for any of things is your plan to fail.

Dr. Wayne W. Dyer in his book, **Your Erroneous Zones**, warns us to put an end to procrastination, to break free from self-destructive patterns, to get out there, and to explore the unknown. Looking at your weekend ahead, in view of the fact you will have more free time, what do you want to do to put yourself first? What would be an accomplishment, putting you, and your weight-loss as a priority?

> *Al: I have an Exercycle that's been sitting there, making a heck of a good clothes rack. I'm going to clean and clear it off, and start using it.*

> *Denise: I'm going to go for a walk on the beach, for me. That's food for the soul.*

> *Robin: I'm going to get into the habit of not watching TV after dinner, but of taking my dogs out for a walk. They'll get some exercise, and so will I.*

Cindy: I plan to buy lots of fresh fruits and veggies, and make homemade soup. Every time I make it, I lose three pounds. My family just loves it, too.

The trick is to make soup from scratch. You will avoid the sodium, processing chemicals and extra calories found in the canned varieties. You will fill up on it, and see a surprising weight loss. Think too, about trying new veggies and recipes to avoid getting bored with the "same-old...same-old."

Another low-fat idea is to serve pasta with added veggies. Your kids won't notice if you sneak ground carrots and broccoli in the spaghetti sauce. Pasta is a food for everyone; it is a happy dish for men, women and kids alike. It's the way to their hearts because it just naturally releases seratonin. Pasta containing wheat or fiber is even better. Try spaghetti squash as a stir-fry, for an interesting new twist.

One little secret, by the way, is to use veggies as a chaser. The idea of "beef in a leaf" is taking something fatty and wrapping it in a veggie, like a dark lettuce. That veggie produces pectin. You may eat something like that and be mystified as to why you would lose weight, especially in light of the fact beef is actually not a good choice, because of all the fat and cholesterol. But beef in a leaf is like wrapping things in jellies and jams; you have seen how they become solidified since they contain pectin, too. In the body, those ingredients bind together, and out they go, along with your fat, along with your high blood pressure, along with any kind of plaque that has been collecting in your system. Of course, a better choice would be to wrap turkey or chicken or fish in a leaf, or even more veggies in a leaf, but the idea is have veggies before, during and after the other things you eat to chase the fat out of your system. Wrap your food in veggies, and you will love what it does for you. As a matter of fact, aim toward eating two and a half to three pounds of veggies a day to help your body find its perfect weight. That's part of putting first things first.

KEY #3: **I**magine yourself slim. sl**I**mmer

Use you imagination to conjure up a vivid picture of the thin you. Visualize every detail. How many pounds do you want to lose? By when? Always have a specific goal in mind. If you have a vague dream, and keep saying, "someday I'll be slim," someday will never come.

However, if you keep focused on your goal with a detailed picture in mind and imagine every aspect of what it will be like to be slim, you will start to notice the benefits you envision. You will experience some big changes. You will have new abilities. You will see dress tags and pants sizes in different numbers. What are some real specifics that you are going for? What are the things you picture daily to motivate yourself?

> *Christy: I want to lose two dress sizes, and feel sexy in a pink bikini.*

> *Annie: I want to look like I did in my wedding picture. I look at it every morning.*

> *Helen: I was always overweight, but now I want to go to my high school reunion, and hear people "ooo" and "ahhh" when I walk in the door.*

> *Al: I want more energy to get my butt off the couch. I picture myself being able to play with my kids one day soon, without huffing and puffing like I do now.*

> *Sarah: For too many years I couldn't climb a flight of stairs without feeling my heart pounding. I've gained more endurance, now that I've lost thirty-five pounds. Now I've made up my mind once I reach my goal weight, I'm going to learn how to rock-climb. That's what I want to do, and by golly, I'm going to do it!*

You know, when you say these things, you move toward them. It's just the way the Universe works. The more you put your BIG dream out there, the closer you come to getting there. Have a sharp vision. Create a clear picture of what you are going to wear. Know what color and style, like Christy's pink bikini. Start clipping out pictures and put these images on your refrigerator. In fact, you might want to think about two pictures. One, which is your most insulting picture you can find of yourself, and another picture of you from a former life, like Annie's wedding picture. Or maybe you'll have to do what I did, since I was like Helen, and had not known what it was to be skinny for quite some time—I clipped a photo out of **Victoria Secrets Catalogue**, and cut-out and glued my face on top of it. I had two pictures, side-by-side for the whole year it took me to lose my sixty-pounds.

Begin with a vivid picture of you at the very end of all your efforts. Where are you going? If you know the answer clearly, you will get there. Dr. Wayne W. Dyer asks us to contemplate the question: "How long are you going to be dead?" Your answer may put your goals in a whole new perspective.

 KEY #4: **M**astermind with others. sli**M**mer

Mastermind with other positive people. Surround yourself with people who cheer you on. Positive people give off positive energy. When you come together with an encouraging person, you create a type of force that equals a whole lot more than just you two. When you come together in support for each other, one plus one equals the strength of eleven. The power created by this mastermind, collectively, gives each person magnetism. It becomes contagious. Sometimes, by hearing other people's tips and successes, and by coming together and being accountable, something is produced with far greater results than any effort you could create on your own.

When I was first battling my weight, I tried to do it on my own. I failed miserably. I couldn't do it. What was missing was the energy I found when I came to my weight support-group meeting each week. Every time I attended, I walked away and saying, "Hey, I can do it—one more pound next week—I can do it!" That came from surrounding myself with upbeat, optimistic people.

You will want to join some sort of support group, too. There are a lot of good ones: Overeaters Anonymous, Slimmons with Richard Simmons, TOPS (Take Off Pounds Sensibly), Weigh Down, Weight Watchers, or any type of group or mastermind to which you become accountable. That is where you will find inspiring people to cheer you on.

Share with your support group of family and friends, as well. The energy you will get from sharing successes with them will help provide you with the sustenance you need to continue your journey to your goal. Besides, when you share your dream, others get attracted to your positive energy. If they have weight to lose, they may become drawn to do what you are doing. You become their role model.

 KEY #5: **M**ake time for you. slim**M**er

Above all else on your calendar, make time for you. Manage your time to ensure you take time-out for you. In the book, *The Seven Habits of Highly Effective People*, Dr. Stephen Covey describes a man working hard at sawing down a tree. He puts forth a lot of sweat and effort, and eventually he gets tired and out of breath.

Someone sees him, and says, "Hey, take a minute to sharpen your saw."

His breathless reply is "I can't—I'm too busy sawing!"

For you, this means sharpening who you are. Would one hour a day be too much? How would you use an hour to become better at who you are? If you dedicate some time to you, you will find every other hour of your day will be far more powerful. You can do this, most importantly, by doing physical exercise. Then, look for more ways to nurture yourself. Look for some wonderful non-food reward to care for your body, mind and spirit. These actions will help you to reach your highest vision. What are some of the things you do to take time for you?

> *Annie: I love to pamper myself in a warm bubble bath. I'm able to just shut out the rest of the world and relax and go within.*
>
> *Christy: I've been listening to motivational tapes when I walk lately. Sometimes I just get so caught up in them, I'll just keep on walking until the tape is over. They cause me to want to aspire higher and higher.*
>
> *Helen: I'm energized whenever I journal. The introspection is so cleansing. I'm much more able to see what I've been thinking. Each time I write, I walk away with a whole new understanding. It's like digging down to get to know myself, and who I am. When I do that, I get to see I do like myself, and that's OK!*
>
> *Al: Reading is my favorite way to re-energize. Lately, I've taken a new interest in nutrition. I've found new revelations. For instance, in today's newspaper I found an article I read about sodium. It was enough for me to tell my wife I'm finally ready to throw away the saltshaker, forever.*

You can see tremendous value in taking time-out for you. Beware. If you get too caught up in your daily "stuff" you lose your efficiency. A lot of people who are overweight are people-servers. They put everyone else first, and as a result, they put themselves last. Remember the instructions you are always given when you fly in an airplane: In the event of an accident, put your oxygen mask on yourself first, before you try to help anyone else.

Don't forget—you can't be of value to anyone else, unless you value yourself. Each day, take your time-out for you.

KEY #6: **E**xpand your mind. slimm**E**r

Expand your mind to be open all people and all things, including yourself. Be non-judgmental. Never say *"never!"* When you expand your mind in this manner, it will bring new acceptance that is very freeing. Try new foods. Be open to all vegetables of the universe. Be open to seek new exercise and adventure. Expand your mind to read new books. Be non-judgmental toward others' methods of weight loss (or weight-gain). Try to appreciate each other, but at the same time, search out available facts and data, which is often the key.

> *Sandra: I have a friend who just can't bear to exercise or to give up fattening food choices. I told her I'm doing something now to help me later on in life. If I can lose twenty or thirty pounds, I know I'll be in good health, and I'll be able to do more later in my life, as a result. I certainly consider that a positive, yet I can't convince her.*

Sometimes our friends don't comprehend, as we do, how important it is to keep a positive frame of mind. Sandra, I know you have done some homework in order to gain insight on how to get the best and healthiest weight-loss results. If your friend could also research, as you have, or listen to what you have learned, she will gain knowledge of fruits and veggies that are going to benefit her health and help her to find her ideal weight. She will discover how vegetables can be used as a "chaser" for the things she is craving. If she could come to the appreciation time spent in exercise is time well invested, because of the quality of life it gives back—she may eventually want the same goals you have.

Unfortunately, that may never happen. As a result, it is important to come to a place where you have patiently heard each other's reasoning, and then do what you know is best for you. I have a friend who swears by a controversial diet, which allows him to eat plenty of fats, but very little vegetables or carbohydrates. He has lost forty pounds, and is convinced he is using the best approach. I have pointed out a diet with so much fat is not sensible, and has been found unsafe by the American Dietetics Association. He, on the other hand, points to studies found in his particular diet book, stating otherwise, and will entertain nothing, other than what he is doing. As a result, we have both listened to each other, we are still good friends, and this is one area where we agree to disagree.

The need to have someone else's agreement is not necessary to our happiness. We don't need others' approval. For many of us, such a concept involves a whole new thinking process.

Frequently people say, "I just can't lose weight," and I find they don't understand, or want to understand what it takes. They may need to do some reading and gain some knowledge. Before that happens, however, they have to desire to change—as much as they would want water in a desert. It may take a defining moment to propel them forward for that to happen. For me, that moment was when I saw a photo that reminded me how much I had gotten to look like my mother who, incidentally, died of weight-related causes. Unfortunately, sometimes that moment never happens. This may explain why obesity is the second leading-cause of death.

Each of us is different from each other, so each of you has different things happening in your metabolism. I, personally, do best with five small meals a day. My husband requires three square meals a day. I require a lot of volume; whereas, he does well with less food than I do. We're all different, and we need to know those differences, in order to make headway.

Each individual also has a pattern. Every fourth week or so, some weight fluctuation occurs, which may be caused by fluid retention and elimination patterns in the body. I have found this to be true of both women and men. This little-known fact is another reason why we need to understand our bodies. It also reminds us to have more patience with ourselves, if we see a periodic gain.

Sometimes we need to talk with the people closest to us and try to work with them, rather than against them. You may have a husband like I do, who wants his hamburgers and French fries. How do you live with him? You'll want to hear him first, to find out where he is coming from, and then seek to have your needs understood, so you can get his support, and still have a winning situation.

I found my husband's cravings for hamburgers could be satisfied with a grilled veggie burger piled high with condiments, tomatoes and lettuce. I also found a wonderful way to make French fries which I brush with egg whites and bake in the oven. Otherwise, we are like two people in the same car, where one wants the windows open, and the other requires the windows closed. So the dialogue goes: "Open!" "Shut!" "Open!" "Shut! And no one gets anywhere. An equal solution for both of us would be to open a vent or a window in the back seat.

So what do you do about the person you live with who needs that fattening something—the very thing that would do you in? Maybe there is a compromise you can work out. Has anyone found a solution?

> Sherrie: *My husband likes his meat and potatoes, too, so now, he has a very large lunch with all the things I would never choose, while he is at work. Then, at dinnertime, together we eat some of my healthier choices. That way, I don't end up being tempted by the rich foods he so loves. So I understand him, and he understands me, too.*

 KEY #7: **R**espond to your weight. slimme**R**

Respond to your weight. Hold yourself accountable. Richard Simmons, America's Fitness Guru, has a great affirmation about accountability. He says, *"I am the one who puts the*

fork in my mouth." When we decide to work on excess weight, we are holding ourselves accountable. We act with responsibility in that we take action.

Highly accountable people are able to look at themselves if they are overweight and say, "I can do it!" "I'm responsible— I am able to take my weight and respond to it."

On the other hand are those who say: *"I can't."*
"I can't do it."
"I can't lose weight."
"I can't exercise."
"I can't get with it."
"I can't eat vegetables."
"I can't drink water."
"I can't write down what I eat."

All those negative people live in a land of *"I can't."* The above are irresponsible statements, spoken as though the weight problem were not their problem. Harvey Mackay in his book, **Swim With the Sharks,** says it well: *"You can't solve a problem unless you first admit you have one."*

I used to say, *"I can't lose because my mother and grandmother were overweight...it's in my genes."* That was a "victim" attitude. I was not being accountable for my own weight difficulty. Come and join me a moment, for a walk in the past:

> I'm a child, waking to a sunny summer Saturday morning in my lace-curtained bedroom, in Milwaukee, Wisconsin. The smells and sounds of sizzling bacon lure me out of bed. I slide into my slippers and plod downstairs to the smoke-filled kitchen, to see Mom standing back from a spitting, black, wrought iron skillet. She magically shrinks a pound or more of the fatty strips, into shiny, crunchy ribbons. Dad bends over the toaster, slathering butter and mayonnaise onto slices of toast. Mom spears several fatty, crispy pieces from the frying pan, and lets them drizzle on top of each piece of bread. Next come the eggs. She cracks them

into the inch-thick grease, as they bubble and pop, forming light, crispy-browned edges. Ladles of fat are poured over the eggs, and plopped onto the bacon-covered toasts.

"Jeannie-gal, sit down, you're just in time," Dad greets me, as he hands me a generous serving.

"Yum!"

"After you eat everything on your plate, we have jelly-filled donuts and coffeecake with sugared-butter crumbles," Mom encourages.

And so it went:

"What's for lunch?"
"Toasted cheese sandwiches, with mayonnaise and bacon. Finish that, and you can have ice cream."
"What about snack?
"Milk and cookies."
"How about dinner?"
"It's Saturday, you know what that means."
"Oh, yeah, steak, pork chops and potato-hush-puppy night."
"...And if you clean your plate, we have your favorite—peanut butter dream bars."

I was brought up that way—I didn't know any other. Our kitchen cupboards were always stocked with a five-pound can of Crisco, a jar of Skippy, a box of Velveeta, and a package of Oreos. Do you identify with this? Funny thing—I remember incredibly few fresh fruits or vegetables. Other parts of my Midwest heritage included: bratwurst, beer, and haystacks of fried onion-rings. Almost everything was served fried (and battered), with plenty of sauce, cheese, butter and salt. Best were the Friday night fish fries—with an abundance of tartar sauce, French-fries, gooey coleslaw, and apple pie.

...And on and on it went. The habits I learned as a child, continued into my adult years. I fed my children the same fare. I puffed up like my mother and grandmother, as I continued to pack on the pounds. By the time I decided to face my weight problem, I was sixty-pounds overweight. I would say, "I can't, lose weight, it's in my genes." Right? Wrong. After looking more closely, I found what was passed-on from generation-to-generation, were not fat genes, but fat habits. Heredity certainly played a factor in contributing to my predicament, but I am happy to report I have broken the mold, and so can you.

We can break the pattern because there is the land of "I can." We can be part of that group of highly efficient people—the people who say, "I am accountable. "I am responsible" "I am able to respond." (Dear reader, I want to let you know this chapter is an adapted transcript from a lecture I gave for weight-loss support. The dialogue that follows here allows you to eavesdrop on the answers to my questions.)

So, what's on your list of actions that shows you hold yourself accountable?

> *Cindy: Journaling. I write down everything I eat. That action keeps me accountable for everything I put in my mouth. If I forget to write something down or take on the attitude of "I'll do it later," my way of thinking gets worse.*

> *Al: I try to drink a half-gallon of water a day. It keeps me from munching and snacking, and curbs my appetite. Also, every day at 3 p.m., I'll have an apple, instead of a Snickers bar.*

Water creates healthy skin, shiny hair, and acts as an aide to digestion. Your habit of drinking six to eight glasses of water daily, gives a tremendous boost to weight loss.

> *Maryann: Exercising is making me more accountable for my weight. I'm finally getting into a responsible habit, so if I don't exercise, I miss it. It's a practice I want to keep for the rest of my life. It's made a big difference in my weight-loss and in my health. I*

dedicate forty-five minutes a day, and it has changed my life.

Robin: I'm doing more positive self-talk. I am able to make responsible choices for my weight loss. I tell myself, "I can get up fifteen minutes earlier and exercise." "I can say 'no' to a second serving of pizza." "I can get in six or more glasses of water a day." I think I was always an "I can't" person before, but now I've got my head on straight.

So, how do you get to be highly effective at weight-loss? If you practice these seven keys daily, you will be a "Highly Effective" loser, and that makes you a real WINNER!

Remember to be **SLIMMER:**
- **S** ee hope. (Think benefits. Think: "I can DO it!")
- **L** ist priorities. (Do first what is most important, and put yourself as first on the list.)
- **I** magine yourself slim. (What do you look like? See it.)
- **M** astermind with others. (The energy of one plus one equals far more than two.}
- **M** ake time for you. (Take time to re-energize. All your efforts will be enriched.)
- **E** xpand your mind. (Listen first, and people will support you.)
- **R** espond to your weight. (You and only you are responsible for your weight.)

Remember, it takes only twenty-one days to break a bad habit, and form a new one to take its place. Start now. You can change your life in less than a month. Taking one small step sets you in motion. The journey of a thousand miles begins with a single step. Do that today. Just say, "I can"!

Read the next chapter right away. You'll be glad you did, because you will discover the POWER of four little words...

 **Chapter Eight**

"I Can Do It!"

"If you think you CAN, you're right!
If you think you CAN'T, you're also right!"
~Henry Ford~

Be your own cheerleader or coach—use affirmations. Affirmations are powerful statements you say to yourself. They are always positive and lift your spirits, (as opposed to negative self-talk, which damages the very fiber of your soul). Think about using affirmations as a way to bolster your self-esteem and encourage yourself. Your inner-voice is constantly chattering. Why not change that self-conversation into supportive dialogue? By making reassuring declarations you boost your confidence and verify your goodness as a capable and worthy person.

I know many people with weight problems are people servers, and put their own needs last. This deprivation often results in weight gain and poor self-esteem. However, remember what you are instructed to do on an airplane. In the case of an emergency, you are taught to put on your own oxygen mask first, before you can take care of the needs of others. In life, you must learn to put yourself first and take time for you, before you can be any help to others.

Affirmations can and do bring about life-changing behavior. If you believe in yourself, you can achieve anything. Below are some proclamations to announce to yourself everyday. You can re-program your thought pattern. With each affirmation, either say it silently to yourself, or say it out loud—but say it with passion. Try to believe each statement. See yourself as though you really own it. Try to visualize yourself doing these things with enthusiasm. With each declaration, stop and tell yourself WHY this affirmation is important to you, and HOW it is working in your life.

At your next opportunity, make a tape recording of your own list of affirmations. Play some of your favorite relaxing music as a background to the tape. Then listen to it as you drive, or walk or exercise. Hearing your own voice will have an amazing effect on your determination to reshape your body mind and spirit. Affirmations help to create BIG dreams. Dare to be great! Here's a start:

- I am awesome.
- I love myself.
- I love how I feel when I love myself.
- I alone am responsible for my life.
- I am the one who holds my fork.
- If it is to be, it's up to me.
- I enjoy working on myself.
- I have specific and measurable goals.
- To reach my goals, I know how I would like to see myself— and what will be different.
- My goals are positive, within my control and a good fit with my life.
- My goals ignite my passion.
- I visualize my goals every day.
- I visualize my goals as complete and achieved—now.

- I have a list of all my goals, which I carry with me.
- I review my goals often.
- I set bigger and bigger goals, as I achieve them.
- I take action on my goals every single day.
- My goals are balanced, and bring balance to my life.
- I create affirmations for all of my goals.
- I say my affirmations every single day.
- I expect to reach my goals.

- I am a peak performer.
- I do whatever it takes, and THEN SOME, in order to achieve my goals.
- If I ever fall off my horse, I get right back on again.
- I tell myself: "It's not what I did, but what I do NEXT that counts."
- I can do anything I choose to do.
- I deserve the best of life.
- I like myself.

- This is my life, and I'm going to live it.
- I am the architect of my life.
- I want to be all that I can be.
- I enjoy spending quiet time with myself.
- In the silence I recharge my batteries and find new energy.
- I do not accept the unacceptable.
- I do what works, and I eliminate what doesn't work.

- I am successful.
- I am terrific.
- I take time to look terrific.
- When people ask me how I'm doing, I respond, "terrific."
- I only do the most terrific things.
- My journey of a thousand miles begins with a single step, which I take today.
- I love to exercise.
- I deserve to exercise.
- I make a date each day with myself to exercise.
- My diet will take my weight off; my exercise will keep it off.
- My exercise produces my energy.
- I sit less; I move more.

- I am enthusiastic and alive.
- I give off energy.
- I radiate aliveness.
- With my unstoppable energy, I easily embrace my goals.
- I wake up early each morning with a smile on my face.
- I look forward to each day, which I start with exercise.
- Each morning I say: "Today is my best day yet."

- I am my best friend.
- I treat myself like my greatest and best friend.
- I praise and applaud myself as I would my best friend.
- My life is happy and rewarding.
- I like smiling, and I smile repeatedly.

- I really believe in the power of my affirmations.
- If I believe it, I will achieve it.
- If I believe it, I will see it.
- I am a "can do," "take action" individual.
- Every day in every way, I am improving.
- I glow with good health and abundant energy.

- I am excited about life.
- I deserve the very best.
- I feel good about myself.
- I am confident.

- As I let go of old baggage and clutter from my life, my energy increases.
- I know what I want out of life, and I go for it.
- I am thankful for a life that is good.
- I laugh easily and a lot.
- I am optimistic.
- I always see my glass as half-full, and never half-empty.
- I am having fun.
- I love my body and treat it well.
- I always have the time to take good care of myself.
- I always have the energy to take good care of myself.
- I always have the desire to take good care of myself.
- I always try to look my best, and I deserve to take time to make sure I do.
- I always wear what makes me look my best.

- On a scale of 1-10, anything I can't grade as a 7 or better does not belong on my body.
- Today is all mine. I go forward with unstoppable energy and confidence.
- I am enthusiastic and eager.
- I love life.
- I am happy.
- I have an abundance of high self-esteem.
- Every way and every day, I raise my self-esteem.

- I am enough.
- I am loveable.
- I am capable.
- I am loving.
- I am loved.
- I am free to be the person I have always wanted to be.
- Every day I become more and more successful.

- I am aware that my thoughts create my world.
- I chose to hold only thoughts that will nurture me.
- I say only positive things to myself.
- I strive to improve myself.
- I take pleasure in improving myself.
- I can do whatever I set my mind to do.
- I always anticipate the best outcome.
- Everyday I become more of the person I want to be.

- I love and accept myself just the way I am.
- I deserve to have my dreams come true.
- I take good care of my body.
- I eat only those foods that are good for me.
- I enjoy tremendous energy because I eat healthy food.
- I have a slim, fit beautiful body.
- I accept my body as it is, and I work to make it even healthier.
- I take time for myself every single day.
- I have a lifestyle that generates high energy.
- I feel freedom in being myself.
- I use my time in ways that fulfill me.
- I believe my needs are as vital as anyone else's.

- I ask for what I want.
- I surround myself with happy, positive and successful people.
- I recognize all those who assist me.
- I am grateful for all the support I receive.

- I move confidently through life.
- I am flexible and easy-going.
- I need only to be myself to get what I want.
- I am open and receptive.
- I easily accept compliments.
- The more receptive I am, the more compliments I receive.
- I easily forgive myself, and get on with my life.
- I choose only that which is for my highest good.
- I have many talents and positive qualities.
- I am pleased with myself

- I seek quality first.
- I seek to know myself.
- It's not what happens that counts; it's how I choose to react to what happens.
- My reactions to what happens make the quality of my life.
- I get into action easily.
- People like me, and that's because I like me first.
- I am responsible for my life.

- I do what makes my heart sing.
- I enjoy doing everything I do.
- I start each day with complete excitement and renewal.
- I do what needs to be done at all times.
- I listen to my inner voice.

- When I chose to act, my fears disappear.
- I experience great satisfaction in completing things.
- I am willing to do what I need to do to succeed.
- I give myself permission to make mistakes.
- I always learn from my mistakes
- I say "no" to those things that take me off purpose.
- I easily say "no" whenever I need to.
- I easily ask for whatever I want.

- I keep on getting better everyday.
- Life is an exhilarating adventure.
- I enjoy the support of many people, and I thank them frequently.
- I learn from the outcomes of my actions.
- I make corrections whenever necessary.
- I am open to feedback.
- I invite comments from others.

- My persistence is fueled by my passion.
- I grow happier and more peaceful every day.
- I reward myself with wonderful non-food rewards for each small success.
- Nothing tastes as good as thin feels.
- If I desire a craving, I will wait fifteen minutes and then decide.
- I think first: "a moment on my lips, but forever on my hips."
- I ask: "on a scale of 1-10, is this craving worth a 10?"
- I tell myself: "it's not a treat; it's a cheat."
- I remind myself: "If I eat right today, I'm a success today."
- I repeat: "if I eat it today, I will wear it tomorrow."

- I am doing everything I can to make my world a better placc.
- I lead an extraordinary life.
- What I make of my life is up to me.
- I have all my tools I need. What I do with them is up to me. The choice is mine.

- It's not the cards I have been dealt, but how I play my hand that really counts.
- To win, first, I must first build a winning hand.
- I choose what will make me feel like a winner.
- It's not on luck or chance I can lay the blame. I must choose my action steps to win.
- I can snack my way to my goal weight, if I pick something sensible, and nutritious.
- I can choose to be more aware and accountable.
- Success lies literally in the palms of my hands.

- If I pay a lot in time and effort, I will receive something far more valuable.
- I am doing this for myself, but not by myself.
- I will not mistake thirst for hunger.
- I will not always be perfect, but I will stick with it.
- It is impossible for me to smile on the outside without feeling better on the inside.
- I will not confuse comfort with happiness.
- I can turn the impossible into two words: I'm possible.
- I can live the thinner life now by daydreaming of the thinner me.

- I watch out for denial and self-sabotage.
- I want this new life for me. I know I am capable of achieving it.
- I believe I deserve it.
- I change all negative self-talk into positive messages.

- I know "stressed" is really "desserts" spelled backwards.
- I focus on how far I've come, not how far I have yet to go.
- I motivate myself by hearing what people will say about the new me.
- I can picture what the new me will look like.
- I can feel what the new me will feel like.
- I learned from my "defining" moment, when I decided I wanted to change.
- I have had many successes in my life. I draw from them, and losing weight is easy.

- I put myself first.
- I take time for hobbies.
- I take time to read and meditate.
- I take time to exercise.
- If I fail to plan, I am planning to fail.
- I have a plan.
- I eat when I am hungry; I stop when I am satisfied.
- I capture my own sense of victory and empowerment.
- I focus on how far I've come. I use these moments to motivate the thinner me.
- I am determined to never gain my weight back again.

- I constantly catch myself wearing a smile.
- My reflection in my mirror shows a posture that reflects a great attitude.
- I try one new veggie each week.
- To change the footprint of my body, I must change the footprint of my mind.
- Some of my biggest obstacles have turned to be my greatest blessings.
- My success is a journey, not a destination.
- I always have another choice.
- The me I see is the me I'll be.

The following affirmations were adapted from a list by "Century 21" Real Estate Company:

I know I am a Winner *(not a Loser)* because:

- I want to win; a loser wants to lose.
- I say, "let's find out;" a loser says, "Nobody knows."
- I say, "I was wrong;" a loser says, "It wasn't my fault."
- I go through a problem; a loser goes around it, and never gets past it.
- I say, "I'm good, but not as good as I ought to be." A loser says, "I'm not as bad as others."
- I try to learn from my superiors; a loser tries to tear down those who are superior to him.
- I look for a better way to do it. A loser says: "that's the way it's always been done here."
- I ask questions and listen to the answers; a loser never listens.
- I discuss opportunities; a loser complains about problems.
- I welcome taking a risk to meet a challenge; a loser won't take a risk.
- I have plans and goals that can be measured. A loser hates measurements.
- I keep statistics; a loser doesn't want statistics.
- I set goals daily; a loser doesn't know what goals are.
- I am not nearly as afraid of losing as a loser is secretly afraid of winning.
- I seek out other winners; a loser seeks out other losers.

The following affirmations were taken from the **Harmony "Prosperity Laws:"**

- I trust that my inner guidance will lead me to my dreams.
- I like who I am and who I am becoming.
- I move ahead at an accelerated pace.
- I see myself as a success.
- I am generous with myself and others.
- Doing what I love serves others.
- My life has purpose and meaning.
- I fully intend to realize my dreams.
- I feel and act as if what I want is already so.
- What I concentrate on expands.
- I mentally release what I no longer want.
- I seek approval from within.
- I believe in myself and my unlimited potential.
- I have an attitude of gratitude.
- I am a forgiving person. (Especially of myself.)
- I am ready and willing to change.

Affirmations DO work. Look at yourself in your mirror several times each day and repeat at least a dozen encouraging thoughts, preferably out loud. Pump yourself up. Write down your favorites and scatter them around your home. Post them on your mirrors and refrigerator. Put them on note cards and carry them in your purse or briefcase. Say them aloud throughout the day. Love yourself enough to try this powerful technique. It will bolster your ego and strengthen your resolve to reach your dreams.

Don't miss the next chapter. Learn things often kept hidden or unexplained. Uncover the mysteries when you discover...

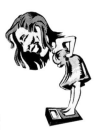

Chapter Nine

"Skinny Jean's" Secrets

DO SOMETHING NOW.
If you have been thinking about losing weight, just get started. Procrastination can last a lifetime. How bad does it have to be before you take action? I remember getting heavier and heavier, year after year, AND it just got worse. When I surpassed my husband's weight, I went into complete denial. I never weighed myself again for an entire year. I needed to take action.

PICTURE YOUR "WAKE-UP" MOMENT.
Go back to your moment of decision that transformed everything. Ask yourself: "What made me finally decide to lose weight?" For me, it was that moment when I saw an embarrassing photo that made me look old enough to be my own mother. For you, it may have been the time you had to lay on your bed and struggle to zip up your pants, or perhaps one day someone asked if you were pregnant (and

you weren't!) Whatever your moment was for you, use it to strengthen your resolve to lose weight right now.

INDULGE IN NON-FOOD REWARDS.

I had to learn to stop my going to food for comfort—something I had done after the trauma of losing five dear people in my family, in a very short period of time. First, I lost my Dad to a very painful death due to cancer. Next, I lost two brothers to AIDS, and then another brother to suicide, and then my Mom, who died of a blood clot—but I think she really died of a broken heart. At the time, Mom couldn't talk of what caused the deaths, so instead of saying it was AIDS, she called it cancer, and instead of saying "suicide," she called it a "Gunshot Wound."

I had my own way of not dealing with the pain. I stuffed down my food, along with all my sorrow, guilt and anger, in hopes my feelings would disappear. What I really needed was to get it out—express my emotions, talk to a friend, put into words the inner turmoil within me. But instead, food became my friend, and my weight began to increase rapidly. I finally learned—if there is a hole in your heart, you could never stuff it with food. Since then, I have learned to turn to some nonfood comforts, and rewards, like calling a friend, going for a walk, taking a warm bath, writing in my journal, or indulging in the wonderful "retail therapy"—shopping!

SAY TO YOURSELF: "THIS IS MY LAST TIME!"

Success came for me during my fourth attempt to lose weight. If you keep losing your same pounds over and over, it's time to get REAL about fat, or—settle on getting really FAT! Face your issues and check your habits. How are you USING and ABUSING food?

SAY TO YOURSELF: "I AM MY SOLUTION!"

When I was overweight, I was unable to see I was responsible for what was happening. I thought maybe my fat would just go away on its own. It's easy to blame our situations on anything and everything but ourselves. If you say, *"I can do this,"* you can, and if you say *"I can't,"* well then...you CAN'T!

JOIN A SUPPORT GROUP.
When I tried to lose weight alone, I failed miserably. It wasn't until I attended a support group regularly that I found the accountability and inspiration I needed to keep me motivated.

KNOW WHAT YOU WANT.
How much do you want to lose? By when? What size do you want to be? What health benefits will you get when you lose your weight? What personal benefits will you experience as you raise your self-esteem? Make a long list. Make it strong enough to peak your desire to lose your necessary weight.

SET A GOAL.
The difference between your daydream and your goal is a DEADLINE. When will you lose ten percent? (Usually in nine to twelve weeks.) When will you drop your next five pounds? Where will you be in your journey a month from now? Six months from now? A year? These are your goals. Without deadlines, you will continue to say: "Someday, I'm going to get skinny."...And someday never arrives.

CHANGE YOUR IMAGE OF YOURSELF:

- **SEE THE NEW YOU.**
Can you picture yourself at your ideal weight? Visualize the new you. Try to really SEE it. What are you wearing? Get a view of the color. Envision the style. See in your mind's eye, the garment tag that tells what size clothing you are wearing. Close your eyes and actually perceive that number. Picture yourself standing on your scale. Visualize that number, as well.

- **HEAR WHAT PEOPLE WILL SAY.**
Close your eyes and HEAR all the things people will be saying about you, when you reach your goal. Picture yourself coming down a long staircase, and listen to all the flattering things they are saying about you. Take note of their faces as they look at you admiringly.

- **TRY TO FEEL YOUR NEW BODY.**

Imagine how it will FEEL when you get to your goal. Visualize your sensation of being able to slide right into your new skinny clothes. Picture your thrill of being able to bend over with ease, to leap up your stairs. Conjure up your pride and satisfaction you will feel in being thin. Can you remember a time when you felt healthiest? Were you a child, a teenager, or was it only a few years ago?

WELCOME A NEW LOOK.

Try a new hairstyle. Or try a different hair color, a dazzling lipstick or a fresh something to note the fact "the new you" has already emerged. Get clothing that is stylish and fitting. Consider having an entire "re-do." You will be marking a new chapter, one that is visibly evident to you. Watch your self-esteem soar. Stay open-minded, and welcome forward-thinking thoughts. This is your time for the new YOU.

RANK YOUR CLOTHES 1 THROUGH 10.

Put a "post-it" on each item of clothing in your closet. If you cannot give it a 7 or more—get rid of it! Wear your most flattering clothes in your best colors. You want to look smashing. No more drab or dowdy stuff—no more muumuus. Get rid of anything that doesn't fit and feel like an absolute dream. Clean out your clutter and make room for the NEW YOU.

NEVER SAY "NEVER."

Never say, "I would never eat that!" (You may.) Or, *"I would never do that!"* After I lost my weight, I found myself considering many new foods, and trying new activities I had never thought I was capable of doing before, because I was carrying around too much weight. Now, I enjoy scuba diving, swimming and long bike rides. I am also thinking someday, I may try skydiving.

DON'T BEAT YOURSELF UP.

Avoid negative self-talk. If you "fall off your horse," so what! Just get right back on. If you lose a dollar, do you throw away your wallet? Never allow disapproving dialogue with yourself. Saying things like *"how stupid of me!"* Or *"I'm such a klutz,"* are destructive to your own self-esteem. Learn to like and love yourself, just the way you are now, and, at the same time, seek to be your best self.

ENJOY YOUR JOURNEY.

Be present in the moment. Losing your weight is half your fun. Record your progress and love yourself now. You are a work in progress. You are in the process of becoming slim.

POST AFFIRMATIONS EVERYWHERE.
Tell yourself things like: *"I can do it!"* *"1 pound by next week!"* *"Size 10 by February!"* or *"I love exercise!"*

YOUR POSTURE = YOUR ATTITUDE.
YOUR ATTITUDE = YOUR POSTURE.

If you smile on the outside, it's impossible to feel bad on the inside. Be an actor, and start with a positive posture, big smile, and unstoppable look of confidence on your face. If you do this, you can just start to feel the same positive confidence and happiness inside. Conversely, if you slouch over, or take on the posture of someone who is tired, or suffering from low self-esteem, you will find it practically impossible to feel happiness on the inside. So, take on your physical characteristics of happiness, and you will automatically feel happy.

THINK OF ANOTHER SUCCESS...ANCHOR TO IT!

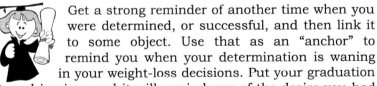 Get a strong reminder of another time when you were determined, or successful, and then link it to some object. Use that as an "anchor" to remind you when your determination is waning in your weight-loss decisions. Put your graduation tassel in view, and it will remind you of the desire you had to complete what you needed to do. That same desire is what you need now, when you find it difficult to keep your food journal. Touch your wedding ring when you are faced with buffet-table goodies, and it will remind you that you were committed to a spouse all these years, and it will take you back you to your commitment you have now to your weight loss. Poke your finger on the back of your earring

and it will remind you to breathe slowly, when you are tempted to inhale that pizza. Instead, you will be reminded of how you kept your calm somewhere else.

SECRETS TO CHANGE YOUR LIFE:

LOOK TO ALTER MORE THAN JUST THE PHYSICAL.
Your decision to lose weight can be a springboard to a whole lot of changes. You can motivate yourself to be your best person you can be in other ways, as well. (Weight can be the ONE thing that gets in your way of EVERYTHING!)

TRY TO IMAGINE WHAT WILL HAPPEN...
Dream of all the things that will happen, once you get to your goal weight. It could mean a whole new you on so many levels. In so many ways, you could change yourself—not just physically, but personally, socially, emotionally, spiritually, professionally, and financially.

PHYSICALLY: You feel sexy, beautiful and slim. You are able to accomplish the things of which you merely dreamed. You have energy and abilities to travel, maybe scuba dive, or go mountain climbing.

PSYCHOLOGICALLY: You have a whole new self-image. You take pride in yourself, and how you look and feel. You have tremendous, unstoppable confidence.

PERSONALLY: You find more and more new ways to improve yourself. You are no longer negative, or blaming of yourself or others. You love yourself, and that reflects on everything you do.

SOCIALLY: You seek positive people to support you. People are attracted to you, because you are a positive person.

FINANCIALLY: You rise to your best potential. You find new ways to experience success. You know ways to set goals and how to accomplish your steps to meet those goals.

PROFESSIONALLY: You have the tools to find happiness in the job of your choice, and to rise to the position best for your authentic and unique self.

SPIRITUALLY: You are able to connect with your inner soul. You view your life as being positive, exciting and passionate. You live with passion.

SEEK OUT ACTIVE, POSITIVE PEOPLE.
Like a Girl Scout, you'll want to "Make new friends, but keep the old," but in making new friends, seek the ones who will be supportive to your efforts. Winners seek out other winners. Seek positive people who make you feel good about yourself, NOT those who zap your energy, and make you feel bad and lower your self-esteem. After I lost my weight, I just naturally found myself attracted to people who were active, happy people. I now have new energetic friends who cheer me on in my efforts. I still have my old friends, but I find I spend less and less time with those who make me feel badly or who dwell continually upon the negative.

IT'S OK TO SPEND SOME MONEY ON YOU.
Your investment in your health is the most important investment you'll ever make. Sure, it's a temptation to buy the 99cent burger because it's cheap, but do you want all that cholesterol clogging up your arteries? Tell yourself it's OK to spend a few dollars on something healthier. Let's face it; your few dollars saved will simply be spent later on larger sizes, or worse yet, on your upgraded casket, when you go to an early grave. (Remember, after smoking, obesity is the second major cause of preventable death.)

Tell yourself it's OK to invest in proper exercise shoes, and membership in a gym. It's OK to reward yourself once in a while, with a non-food reward for your progress. It's OK to spend your money on joining a support group. If you don't allow yourself to spend some money now, the amount you save could easily go for doctors, or hospitals, or psychiatrists or medical prescriptions later.

MAKE A STUPENDOUS LIST:

WRITE.
Write your goals. Write the steps you will take
to achieve them. Write why you think you are
capable. Write visualizations of what you will
look like, feel like, and what others will say about you. Write
your dreams and beliefs, and why you believe they can
happen. The best gift I ever got was when I had lost my first
thirty-five pounds, and I was given a journal. I used it to
pour out all the good and positive things in my heart. The
things I wrote helped to motivate me to go my extra twenty-
five pounds to my goal. I wish I had given myself that gift
right from the beginning, because by my writing, I was able
to see more clearly what was just mixed-up spaghetti in my
head.

WRITE FIVE THINGS YOU ARE GRATEFUL FOR DAILY.
My daughter gave me the book entitled **A Simple
Abundance,** by Sarah Ban Breathnach, and it changed my
life. In it, Sarah suggests you write five things you are
grateful for each night before you go to bed. This little
practice has transformed me into a far more positive, loving
and sensitive person. Try it.

LIST THE SPECIFIC THINGS YOU WILL NEED TO DO.
What steps do you need to take to accomplish your goals?
This was MY list:
1. Talk to my family, to ask their support and
   agreement about the foods we will have and not
   have around our house.
2. Go shopping for a specific list of those things that
   will support my efforts.
3. Make a big pot of vegetable soup to snack on when I
   am hungry. (See recipe in this chapter.)
4. Get out my sneakers, and decide on daily exercise.
5. Set my alarm clock a half hour earlier.
6. Pack a "Snack-Attack Survival Kit" for the car and at
   work.

What steps will YOU need to take: Make a list, or draw
stickmen to help you visualize your process.

KEEP TRACK OF YOUR FOOD.

Keep a journal, and write down every bite, lick and taste. If your calorie total goes beyond your daily limit, write it all down, anyway. We all fall off the horse, once in awhile, so it helps you to be accountable, and it may not be as bad you thought. You're learning new habits, and are practicing new choices, without always knowing it. Just know you can "reboot" your computer right now, and you don't have to wait until tomorrow or Monday. What matters is not what you have done, so much as what you do NEXT. I learned to forgive myself, learn from my mistakes, and love myself for making the good choice to start over.

IF YOU BITE IT, YOU WRITE IT.

Write down every taste, lick and nibble. It's so easy to forget a second helping, or that cream in your coffee, or a single cookie. Don't be a "Pinocchio," with your calories, or they will be double without your even knowing.

TELL PEOPLE ABOUT YOUR GOALS.

Telling friends and family you're trying to lose weight, will reinforce your own commitment, and may cause them to join you, as well. Invite them to join you. The biggest mistake I made was keeping my weight-loss efforts a secret. I was so afraid I would fail; I decided I was not going to tell anyone I had joined a support group. It wasn't until I lost my first twenty-five pounds that people started to ask me what had happened. As soon as I told them I had joined a support group, several of them joined immediately. To think I had gone my first half of that journey alone, when I could have shared it with those I cared about most. It was so much more fun to have a few friends there for support. People will get attracted to your goals, and ask you how it's going. What you talk about will begin to manifest itself.

POST A POSITIVE AND A NEGATIVE PICTURE.

Put a picture of what you would like to look like on your refrigerator. If you have never looked like that, then look through catalogues, like *"Victoria Secrets,"* and clip one out. Put your own face on it. Visualize the new you. Next, put your most insulting picture you can find of yourself right next to it. Deliberate which picture you want to look like, each time you open the door to your refrigerator.

SAY: *"THIS IS NOT A DIET, BUT A LIVE IT."*
Tell yourself the habits you are learning will be for a lifetime of healthy living. This is not a quick fix, but something your whole family can do with you, so you can all live long, happy, healthy lives together.

A-S-K IN ORDER TO G-E-T.
Don't be afraid to ask for support. No one knows you need help, unless you make yourself vulnerable and make it known you need his or her help. Be sure to tell that person PRECISELY what it is they can do.

For years I had a problem with always eating the leftovers as I cleared the plates after dinner. What I needed to do was to ask my husband to help support me with my problem of never wanting to waste anything, which stemmed from an old childhood tape in my head—*"think of the poor, starving children in China,"* etc. (Well, I have news—the children in China are now getting FAT!) But it wasn't until I told him how much his support meant to my success, if he would please help me specifically by him being the one to clear the table of leftovers, because I just could not let anything go to waste, or it would go right to my "waist." He was all too happy to help me out, and I wondered why I had never explained this to him, or asked for his help before.

When my bridge club went to our annual "dinner and a play" Christmas celebration, I found it difficult to speak up and ask that we not go to a Mexican restaurant. But I knew if I didn't ask for their support, I might resort to old behaviors, and dive facedown into the chips! They were most gracious in their understanding, and I wondered why I had been hesitant to ask their support for similar events in the past. My prior self-image had been a roadblock for me.

BRING HOME NOTHING THAT WILL SABOTAGE YOU.
Stop disabling yourself and others. Let nothing enter your grocery basket that is not a direct support to your efforts. Tell others if they need candy, chips, ice cream, pizza, or

any of the things you know to be your "Red Light Foods" they will have to bring them home themselves, and to please hide them if they do.

BE A PROLIFIC EATER—OF VEGGIES—THAT IS.
It doesn't matter how MUCH you eat, but rather WHAT you eat. You can eat HORDES of veggies and burn "negative" calories, because your body uses more calories in just trying to digest the extra fiber.

TRY ONE NEW VEGGIE EACH WEEK.
Ever try jicama? How about eggplant or bell peppers and onions on your grill? Try red-beets with a sprinkling of walnuts.

HAVE "EASY TO GRAB" SNACKS ON HAND.
Don't allow yourself to get so ravenous you can't stop that "Halloween Monster" who has awakened within you, that wants to grab at ice cream, or pizza, and other things far less sensible. When you open your refrigerator, have unwrapped, easy-to-reach, finger-foods, like cherry tomatoes, baby carrots or grapes on hand to satisfy you. Carry the same things in your car, so your hunger does not drive you to your nearest fast food restaurant, where to your dismay you hear yourself asking for the "Super-size."

PACK A SANDWICH FOR LUNCH.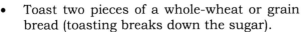
Take time to plan in advance, and you will keep your focus and determination. Try my favorite sandwich:
- Toast two pieces of a whole-wheat or grain bread (toasting breaks down the sugar).
- Spread ¼ avocado (a good fat, if used in moderation), on one piece of the bread.
- Stack the middle high with cucumbers (one of nature's most perfect veggies, because of the water content), tomatoes (a great cancer preventative, and a fat-burner with other foods), and spinach—the leaves lay flat, and are filled with powerful nutrients.
- Use mustard and garlic powder on the other piece.
- After lunch, take time for a walk.

USE SPRAY BUTTER.

No kidding—I carry spray butter with me everywhere. I threw away the butter, margarine and saltshaker I had used so freely. That spray product contains zero sodium, zero fat and zero calories. It is a water and soy product, and has less hydrogenation than margarines, and that's going to help in reducing high blood pressure and cholesterol. My doctor loved the new readings, and I was able to throw away the high blood pressure pills I had used for over twelve years. You will love the flavor, along with your weight-loss. Also, try new spices, like garlic, rosemary, dill, lemon, lime, and whatever has flavor, but is low in sodium.

SERVE SOUP.

Oh, the miracle of soup! I have seen many people lose an initial five pounds or more in the very first week. You can experience a similar weight loss anytime. Just fill up on soup, and feel the nutritional benefits, as well. If it's hot out, serve it cold. If it's cold out, serve it hot. Try new kinds, too. Gazpacho is a great soup for hot weather. Use fresh or frozen ingredients, and stay away from the sodium, processing and extra calories from canned goods.

SKINNY JEAN'S "JUMPSTART" SOUP

3 cloves garlic, minced
4 carrots, sliced
4 onions, chopped
2 cups cabbage, chopped
2 celery stalks, chopped
1 ½ pounds mushrooms, sliced
4 cups fat-free low-sodium broth
2 T tomato paste (no salt added)
1 T dried oregano
½ t dried basil
Freshly ground black pepper, to taste
Minced parsley
Salt substitute to taste (Try "It's a Dilly," or Chef Paul Prudhommene's Magic Seasoning)

1. In a large saucepan, sprayed with nonstick cooking spray, sauté the garlic and onions over low heat until softened, about 5 minutes.

2. Add 1 cup of the broth, along with the carrots and celery. Cook, stirring as needed until softened, 6-8 minutes. Add the mushrooms and cook, stirring as needed, until the mushrooms begin to soften.
3. Add the rest of the broth, along with the cabbage, and seasonings. Bring to a boil, lower heat and simmer, partially covered, stirring as needed, until tender, about 30 minutes.
4. Garnish with parsley and serve. (It tastes even better the next day.)

TRY EATING SOUP FOR BREAKFAST.
Be open-minded. Some homemade vegetable soup will perk you up if you're feeling tired, or sluggish. Eat it all day long. It will fill you up and help you to lose as much as five pounds in a week!

START YOUR DAY WITH A FRUIT SMOOTHIE.
You'll get a lot of energy from fruit or a fruit smoothie, and you'll get in a serving of calcium, besides. I had experienced a frustrating plateau with no weight loss for what seemed like weeks. But then I broke right through that exasperating period by having a smoothie and fruit until noon each day.

Fruit is filling and will curb your appetite. If you don't eat proteins or carbohydrates until noon, you allow your body to continue burning and digesting food from the day before. Meanwhile, you will get the energy you need to start your day. As fruit is digested in about twenty minutes, your system can go back and continue burning yesterday's calories, while you get the benefit of a better weight loss.

TRY BROILED INSTEAD OF FRIED.
Look for healthy words like: "baked," "broiled" or "barbequed." Stay away from fried foods; they're normally full of fat (and calories). Avoid words like: "battered', "buttered," "creamy sauce," as well. Anything that shines usually contains fat, and unhealthful cholesterol.

GROW YOUR OWN SPICES.
Rev up your metabolism with spices. Try the stems from a rosemary bush to skewer fish or make shish kebobs. Plant

some garlic, dill or cilantro. I used to salt everything without even tasting it. Once I started using natural spices, I never missed the sodium, or the way it caused me to bloat.

SOY TO THE WORLD!
I found soy products to be a great way to get my calcium, fight hot flashes and PMS. Since I am a Cancer survivor, soy and tofu are a better choice for me, as a natural hormone replacement. A cup of non-fat soymilk is merely seventy calories, and makes a great base for a morning smoothie. Add some tofu and whatever fruit is in season, and you have a tasty, healthy drink. Some of those nonfat soy burgers are as low as seventy calories, and can make a delicious lunch on a bun, piled high with lots of veggies, catsup and mustard. (Plenty of calories left for later.)

ADD LEMON.
There's a reason why so many oriental people are slender. They garnish their dishes with lemon, which acts as a catalyst to protein and helps to burn fat. Lemon also acts as a zestful addition to your water without the added calories.

TAKE TIME FOR YOU.
You deserve it! Pamper yourself with nonfood rewards, like a relaxing bubble bath, a cup of tea. Take a walk. Meditate. Write. Find and connect with your inner soul.

Now we're going to move to the next step—keeping your weight off. You'll want to read the next chapter where you will learn...

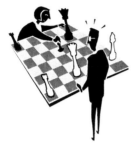

Chapter Ten

"Skinny Jean's" Strategies

Strat-e-gy ('strat-e-je) *noun.* **The art of devising plans toward a goal.**

TRY SOME "STREET-SMART" STRATEGIES:

DON'T GET "WAISTED."
If you are a member of "The Clean Plate Club" and are afraid to waste anything, consider it will go to your own "waste disposal"—your waist. Leaving just a small bite of everything on your plate is one way to prove to yourself you have control over your food, and it is not controlling YOU. Pick up a piece of chocolate cake, or pizza, and run it under your faucet. Watch as it disappears down the drain. Do this at least once, and you will experience an entirely new sensation of control. Give away leftovers, rather than let them tempt you.

TAKE YOUR OWN POPCORN TO THE MOVIES.
Buy popcorn in bulk and pop it in an air-popper, a microwave popper, or put it in a brown paper bag and pop it in the microwave. Then take your own popcorn in a Nordstrom's shopping bag when you go to the movies. Don't

forget your spray butter. No one will stop you or even notice. If they do, be ready to tell them you're ALLERGIC to their popcorn—and you ARE—it makes you BREAK out—in great blobs of FAT! (They prepare it in coconut oil, the deadliest of all fats!)

WEAR A BELT

If I wear a belt, I become more aware of when I eat too much. A belt reminds me to continue to suck-it in and look slim. Try this from the start and you will see you'll be adjusting the notches on that belt tighter and tighter. You'll have a visible record of your progress that is far more rewarding than any tape measure.

ASK YOUR PHARMACIST FOR ANOTHER CHOICE.

Prescription drugs and hormones often cause bloating and weight gain. Because these drugs cause water retention, many perturbed people battle their weight, week-after-week, with little or no progress. They may avoid the excess weight gain, if they ask their pharmacist to suggest the name of a suitable alternative. (Often the pharmacist knows the full range of what is available. The patient can then go back and ask the doctor for the more suitable prescription.) If this cannot be done, perseverance is the only key. People on medication CAN accomplish weight-loss—only it is a lot harder.

DO YOU REALLY WANT CREAM IN YOUR COFFEE? BETTER YET, DO YOU REALLY <u>WANT</u> COFFEE?

When I found out how many calories I had to spend for cream in my coffee, I tried going without it, and found I didn't actually miss it. (I spent the extra calories on foods that absolutely satisfied me.) Then, after losing twenty-five pounds, and hitting a tremendously long plateau of no weight-loss at all, I learned coffee was in fact a detriment to my losing weight. Once I gave it up, I found, once again, the pounds just peeled away.

USE MEAT AS A CONDIMENT.

Meat portions are often the source of weight problems, and should be kept to a minimum. We need protein, but merely about three to four ounces a day. Use meat as a flavoring.

The "main event" should be the vegetables, and meat is a "side dish," or just a condiment. Every dinner should include a salad and a cooked vegetable or two.

PARTIES! PARTIES! PARTIES!

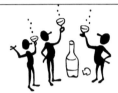

BYOV!
BYOV means **B**ring **Y**our **O**wn **V**eggie dish to share at parties and gatherings. Every hostess will love you. This strategy will keep you from getting tempted by all the party foods normally tempting you. Have a healthy helping of the dish you brought first. Then take a taste of the other foods.

WATER WILL FILL YOU UP.
Drink two glasses of water before arriving at the party. This can be your diet. Instead of alcohol, order a wine "spritzer" (wine mixed with seltzer). Alternate with another glass of water.

DRINK YOUR WATER WITH ICE.
You burn more calories drinking ice water than drinking water at room temperature. Your body works harder to raise the temperature of the water to match that of your body temperature.

CHEW ON ICE.
Chewing ice will give your mouth something to do, and there are no calories, either. (Just be careful not to crack your teeth.)

MAKE A LIST OF PARTY TOPICS.
Social gatherings often mean lots of food, and that means lots of sabotage, unless you are ready with a plan. Visualize yourself talking to many people. Think ahead of time of what you want to know to catch up on their lives. What do you want to have them know about you? Think of some newsy-items, and jokes you can tell.

Arm yourself with attitude. Mentally rehearse how you will move away from the food, and practice in your mind how you will stand, with one hand holding a glass of water, your other in your pocket, etc. Pay more attention to the people, and focus little on the food. Remember, you can always eat when you get home, but you may not get to see these people again for a long time.

AT THE RESTAURANT...

BE ASSERTIVE WHEN DINING OUT
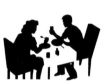
Don't be afraid to ask how something is prepared. Get it "broiled" instead of "fried." Ask for salad dressing "on the side." Then try the "fork trick," and dip only the tines of your fork with dressing. Next, spear your salad to get enough of the taste, but when you finish there should be almost as much dressing left, as when you began. Ask for unbuttered toast (bring your OWN spray, I do.) Ask for egg whites or eggbeaters. Substitute tomatoes for French fries. Leave off the cheese, but DO ask for salsa.

"PRETEND" YOU ARE THIN.
How do thin people do it? Notice them at parties and restaurants. They pick at their food. They eat a skinny piece of pie. They engage more in conversation, rather than focusing on the food. Make believe you are skinny. Check your behavior.

AT HOME...

EAT IN THE NUDE.
Don't laugh. You will be less likely to pig out, if you are conscious of your body. You won't want to eat as much. You will become more aware of that bulging stomach, and all the other things you want to change.

EAT IN FRONT OF A MIRROR.
Try this exercise, and you will be amazed at certain habits and mannerisms of which you will want to be more aware.

ALLOW ENOUGH TIME TO EAT SLOWLY.

Slow down! People often get so hungry from not eating in between meals, they gobble their food at mealtime. Like a dog, they will woof down everything until it is gone. Eating sensible snacks during your day helps to stave off ravenous hunger. Put an index card next to you, at your table where you are eating to remind yourself to:

- Move and eat in slow motion.
- Cut food into tiny pieces
- Savor every bite.
- Put your fork down between each bite.
- Chew food at least twenty times.
- Don't put more food in your mouth until you have completely swallowed your previous bite.
- Take time to really look at and talk to the person with whom you are eating.
- Watch out for the "eat and run" syndrome.

THEY WILL NEVER KNOW.

Pasta is your way to every man and kid's heart. If you have fussy kids, or a spouse who won't eat veggies, just make pasta and spaghetti dishes, and slip in carrots or broccoli into the pasta sauce. They'll never know it, BUT you'll all get healthy together. (Carrots provide a natural sweetener, too!)

USE A SMALL PLATE.

Play some mind games with yourself. A smaller plate will convince you you've had plenty to eat. Also, use a pretty plate, set a pleasing table, complete with candles and fancy water glasses. Add a slice of lemon for a delightful effect. Mealtime will be special, and you will feel pampered. (And, of course, eat only when sitting down. It's so easy to have those extra nibbles while standing up. You will forget, and wonder later why you can't lose weight.)

NEVER SERVE "FAMILY STYLE".

"Family style" allows you to reach for second helpings without even thinking about it. I serve meals "hotel style" instead, and put the pots and casserole dishes on the stove.

That way, I must make a conscious effort to get up and announce to myself: *"I am going for a SECOND helping."* Putting those serving dishes away BEFORE I sit down to eat is an even better alternative.

USE A MAGIC MARKER TO CIRCLE OR WRITE THE CALORIES ON PANTRY AND FREEZER ITEMS.
You'll do it merely once that way, and it will serve as an easy reminder. My ten-year-old grandchild has learned how to look up calories, and loves to do this job for me whenever she comes over.

GET THOSE HANDS OUT OF THE FOOD.
Try some new hobbies if you are a boredom eater. Get those photos out of shoeboxes and into albums. Try a new craft. Cruise the Internet, and you will quickly lose track of time. Try needlecraft or painting. Get so absorbed in a hobby that you forget to eat.

DON'T EAT BEFORE BEDTIME.
If you are tempted to eat a little something before bedtime, just take pleasure in that feeling, and know if your body is hungry, it will use up your stored fat to satisfy the hunger. You will wake up in the morning weighing less, and the hungry feeling will be gone. Not only that, but food in your body at bedtime merely lies there and never gets assimilated because your body is inactive.

EAT ASPARAGUS AND MELON THE DAY BEFORE YOU WEIGH-IN.
Now, here is a tip used by many of my weight support-group staff members, who are required to weigh-in monthly. Like anyone else, they fear the old "fat person" may come back. They often eat asparagus and cantaloupe the day before their weigh-in, as these foods act as natural diuretics.

TAKE A LONG WHIFF OF THE THING YOU ARE CRAVING.
Try it! Smell a candy bar for thirty seconds. You'll be amazed at how you can feel satisfaction thru your olfactory senses, without ever taking a bite.

POSTPONE.
Many times you think you are hungry, when you are actually bored, stressed or lonely. Postpone your cravings for twenty minutes, and do something else, instead. Go for a walk, clean a drawer, make a call or leave the site of the food. After twenty minutes, you may have easily forgotten about your hunger. The remarkable thing is if you tell yourself you may eat that thing sometime later, later may never come.

MAKE IT FUN.
Weight loss can be fun, if you find ways to make it like a game. Chart your progress. Make deals with yourself. Post goals, such as: *"When I lose 5 pounds, I will reward myself with a pedicure."*

EXERCISE STRATEGIES:

SNEAK IN EXTRA EXERCISE.
First, get to know and believe the payback of exercise is enormous and life giving. Then, find more ways to do more. I got great results from doing leg-lifts and leg-lunges while blow-drying my hair, doing my make-up, curling my eyelashes, or talking on the phone. Do something while driving—suck in your tummy, do isometric lifts of one arm or leg at a time. Walk further when going to the store, and meetings. Take the stairs. Welcome extra trips and ways to incorporate more and more steps. Wear a pedometer from morning till night and challenge yourself to do the Federal Government's standard of 10,000 steps a day. (I don't go to bed until I do at least that much, because I am now convinced the time spent in exercise has helped me gain back at least twenty years of youth and vitality.) Exercise should be done as regularly as you brush your teeth. So the next time you brush your teeth, remember to sneak in some exercise.

EMPTY AND FILL YOUR LUNGS COMPLETELY.
Get more oxygen to your body by breathing deeply. You will rev up your metabolism if you try to completely fill and empty your lungs. Try this even as you are driving, or

sitting. Apply this as you exercise, and you will see the results on the scale. Oxygen to your brain increases brain function. Breathing in more oxygen also improves your attitude as you take in more seratonin from the air, which releases mood-lifting endorphins in your brain.

IF YOUR EXERCISE BUDDY DOESN'T SHOW UP, DON'T USE THAT AS AN EXCUSE.

Your exercise should be a date with YOU. You owe it to yourself, and will be richly rewarded by making exercise a habit.

LISTEN TO TAPES.

Music can boost your spirits. Motivational tapes can elevate your soul. Listen to tapes while you exercise, and get twice their effect.

PLAN SOME BAREFOOT WALKS AT LOW TIDE.

If you are fortunate to live near coastal waters, get a tide calendar so that you can plan to walk at low tide. To enjoy this experience to the fullest, do it in your bare feet, and walk at ankle depth. It's a wonderful sensual experience, and may present you with lots of adventure, too. You may find starfish, sand dollars, or perhaps you will see dolphins. Spotting a dolphin may bring you good luck, but more importantly, you have gotten yourself outside to enjoy yourself—through exercise.

DO ARM EXERCISES FROM THE START.

After losing my sixty pounds, I had a big disappointment. My arms had not kept pace with the weight-loss I saw on the rest of my body. I was encouraged when I met a woman who had lost over one hundred pounds whose arms looked great. I asked her for her secret. She lifted weights from the very beginning. I tried the same, and in about eight weeks, I began to see wonderful results. Work on those arms right now, even if it's just with soup cans in your living room. Then, work up to heavier weights, later.

WALK A MILE ON THE PHONE.

A telephone conversation can be an opportunity to exercise. Make every minute count. Multi-task, and you'll burn more calories. If you are stuck with a sedentary day at your office, find ways to add more steps. Get up often, and walk around.

LAUGH A HUNDRED TIMES A DAY.
Laughing, itself, is a great exercise. One hundred good belly laughs a day, over a week, will result in one more pound of weight loss. So, laugh your pounds away!

GET UP A HALF-HOUR EARLIER.
This was one new habit that changed my life. By setting my alarm clock a half-hour earlier, and resolving not to just hit the snooze alarm, again, I found I could get in that exercise about which I had been procrastinating. You will find you burn more calories, if you get less sleep. You will find you need less sleep when you are more active. You'll have time to plan you day—to reflect, and to meditate.

BUY A DOG.

A dog is really an "exercise machine with hair." Besides, a pet is a source of unconditional love. When you feel stressed or down, that wagging tail is always there, just for YOU!

MAKE AN AUDIO TAPE IN YOUR OWN VOICE.
You will be amazed at how hearing affirmations in your own voice can have a magical effect on your weight loss. Make a list of positive messages that mean something special to you, and record them. Play your tape in your car as you drive, or listen on headphones as you exercise.

REMEMBER: YOUR DIET WILL <u>TAKE</u> IT OFF, BUT EXERCISE WILL <u>KEEP</u> IT OFF.
In order to have a life-style change, exercise has to be a high priority. I never look upon exercise as a waste of time, now. The real waste was all the time I spent being fat.

PRACTICE SAYING "NO!"

- **PRACTICE SAYING "NO" TO YOURSELF.**

Strengthen your will power through mental exercise. See the cheese as a mound of fat clinging to your thighs. Try other gross images as well. Would the dessert look half as good if you knew someone spit on it in the kitchen?

- **PRACTICE SAYING "NO" TO OTHERS.**

Managing people who insist you eat can be a difficult task. The pressure to please others can seem immense. But succumbing to those who "bait" you doesn't make you achieve your goals. Keep your goals in mind and have some answers ready as weapons that will protect you. It is all right to admire the beautiful display of food. Making comments such as, *"everything looks so delicious,"* is one way to please the hostess. Sampling small well-chosen foods and setting your limits is critical in managing these stressful situations.

The best exercise to learn is: turn your head quickly, to the left-and-right...left-and-right. It's also a good idea to become skilled at telling a couple of white lies to food pushers who just won't take *"no"* for an answer. Tell them you can't eat another bite...tell them you have a toothache...tell them you feel like you may throw up at any minute, and tell your mother-in-law you will save the cheese cake she made "especially for you" until later. (It's best to rehearse what you will say ahead of time, and practice.)

SOMETHING FOR YOUR BODY:

HANG A BATHING SUIT THAT DOESN'T FIT YET, IN THE FRONT OF YOUR CLOSET.
Let it be bait or a reminder of what you're aiming for. Visualize yourself slim enough to fit into it.

TRY NEW SIZES.
Each time you lose ten pounds, try on a new clothing size, or you may miss the thrill that there is LESS of YOU!

YOU HAVE THE RIGHT TO "BARE ARMS."
It's summer. Show those arms! Don't be ashamed of them. Same thing goes for legs and tummy. Just remind yourself you are a "work in progress!"

MAKE A DATE WITH YOURSELF TO EXERCISE.
Treat your date to exercise as importantly as you would a luncheon date with a friend, or an important business meeting

LOOK FIVE POUNDS THINNER IMMEDIATELY.
Tuck in your shirt, and suck-in my tummy. You will find you not only look slimmer, but you will feel slimmer. You will also strengthen your abdominal muscles, and start to genuinely WANT to lose weight. Don't wear a lot of stretchy things with forgiving waistbands. You will not be aware of your progress, and you'll find they are far too lenient. Get rid of the muumuus-they allow you to go back and visit old chapters to which you'd rather say *"goodbye!"*

SOMETHING FOR YOUR MIND:

TELL YOURSELF: *"I DESERVE TO BE THIN."*

As a weight-loss counselor, I find many people who are excessively overweight have the same pattern of poor self-esteem. They put themselves last, and feel undeserving. I tell them they deserve feeling good just as much as anyone else. I ask them if it were someone in their family who was trying to lose weight, wouldn't they deserve it, and do everything they could to support them, as well?

TELL YOURSELF: *"I CAN BREAK THE MOLD."*
You CAN "kick the can." If your excuse for being overweight is your heredity, it is simply that—an excuse. I have seen hundreds of people who have experienced significant weight loss, who at one time thought FAT was their FATE.

READ SUCCESS STORIES.
Those success stories are about ORDINARY people, just like you. Remember: ordinary people can do EXTRAordinary things—just like YOU!

RECOGNIZE A COMPLIMENT.

When you start to lose your weight, people don't always know what is happening. They may be afraid to ask, for fear they may be insulting you. They may wonder if you are sick. Or they may say things like: *"Is that a new dress you're wearing?"* (And it's one you've worn many times.), or: *"Is that a new hair-style?"* (And it's your same old style you've always worn.) The best compliment I got from my son, after I had lost sixty pounds was: *"Mom, you're getting to look like a runt!"* Hearing those words made my heart sing.

DO IT NOW. SHUT OFF YOUR TV.

Procrastination can often be the very reason you put weight on in the first place! What have you been putting off, and why? When you breakout of old patterns, sometimes, your weight goes with it. One example how we waste time in putting things off is our habit of watching just one more television program. (It is estimated the average person watches sixteen years of TV in his lifetime!)

SOMETHING FOR YOUR SPIRIT:

FILL YOUR HEART NOT YOUR MOUTH.

The next time you are faced with tempting foods, keep your vision of yourself at your GOAL, and tell yourself: *"Nothing tastes as good as THIN feels!"* Go within, and ask your higher power to fill your spirit, instead.

IT'S NOT THE FOOD WE PUT IN OUR MOUTHS.

Sometimes it is the thoughts we put in our heads that do the damage. Our negative self-talk can be devastating, especially after a setback. Instead of forgiving ourselves, and getting right back on program, we lead ourselves into a downward spiral. If God forgives us, we certainly can forgive ourselves. Use positive affirmations to fill yourself and create a bright and shiny spirit. (See the chapter entitled *"I CAN DO IT!"*)

MAKE YOURSELF VULNERABLE.

Don't be afraid to reach out and talk to people when you are hurting. It wasn't until much later, when I finally was able to talk about the secrecy that surrounded the AIDS and suicide deaths in my family that I found others had similar problems, too. It seems that everyone has a family secret hidden somewhere. My being able to talk about my own family allowed others to speak about their own pain as well. You may find what you share will help liberate others, and helping them will make your spirit soar.

GET A MENTOR, BE A MENTEE.
Find someone whom you admire, who was successful at losing weight. Try to model that person. You can also benefit from helping others with pointers you have acquired in your weight-loss journey.

TAKE YOUR "ROCKING CHAIR" TEST.
Ask yourself now—when you are ninety-five years old in your rocking chair, what will you regret not doing? What will be your answer? What things have you dreamed of doing, but were stopped by your weight? Will you regret, as I did, never learning to scuba dive? Want to travel to Greece, but you know you cannot climb all those stairs? Maybe you always dreamed of learning to sky dive. Or perhaps you'd like to go hiking or biking...try a new career...learn a new language...or?

DON'T EVER MISS YOUR SUPPORT GROUP MEETING.
Once I finally got focused, I attended every meeting, even if my weight was up, for those were the times I found attending most important. Remember, it doesn't matter so much what you have done. So what, if you have blown it— it's what you do NEXT, that counts. Going to the gathering will help give you the support you need to re-strengthen your focus and visualize your goals, once again. Meetings help empower your positive belief about yourself. You will see others lose weight, and it will let you know there's nothing special about them—if THEY can do it, so can YOU!

GET THE "SKINNY" ON THESE TIPS:

BE PATIENT.
You didn't put your weight on all at once, so it won't come off all at once, either. A pound a week is all I ever saw. It

took me a year to lose my sixty pounds, but a year passes anyway, and "Viva La Difference!" I know I got back at least twenty-years in youth, vitality and quality of life.

RE-READ THESE TIPS.
Review these tips, and this entire book, over and over. Keep them in your bathroom, or at your bedside. Months from now, you will find you are learning something new in a different way. You will experience a deeper understanding.

START BINGING ON LIFE.
Are you using food as a substitute for REALLY living? Use your weight-loss as a catalyst for all kinds of changes. Be open to new things, people, and activities. Reshape your body, mind and spirit. Call upon the POWER of Spirit within you right now. Be:

- **P ositive**
- **O pen**
- **W illing**
- **E nthusiastic**
- **R esponsible**

Sometimes you may be afraid to dream because you are afraid you might fail. Or you may be afraid of your own success and what it may mean—possible loss of relationships or additional responsibilities. You may fear what others may think. What comes out of success may be too much for you to handle. You may fear you can't do it alone. Whatever your fear, remember, you are never alone. You have the power of Spirit. To call upon that power, you need only go within. When you do, you are "POWER LIVING." You will aspire to all that Our Divine Creator has seen for you. You will reshape your body, mind and spirit. You will surely live your BIG dreams. You will liberate yourself to be brilliant, gorgeous, talented, fabulous and skinny because...

OUR DEEPEST FEAR

Our deepest fear is not that we are inadequate.
Our deepest fear is that we are powerful beyond measure
It is our light, not our darkness
that most frightens us.
We ask ourselves, who am I
to be brilliant, gorgeous, talented and fabulous?
Actually, who are you not to be?
You are a child of God.
Your playing small doesn't serve the world.
There is nothing enlightened about shrinking
So that other people won't feel insecure around you.
We were born to make manifest
the glory of God that is within us.
It's not just in some of us; it's in everyone.
And as we let our own light shine,
We unconsciously give other
people permission to do the same.
As we are liberated from our own fear,
our presence automatically liberates others.

by Marianne Williamson, Author, **A Return to Love.**

...And so, Dear Reader, I ask you: Why the wait?
WHY THE WEIGHT? Dare To Be GREAT!

Best wishes to a **NEW** you,

Jean Krueger

BIBLIOGRAPHICAL REFERENCES

Adams, Rex. *Doctor's Amazing Speed Reducing Diet.* West Nyack, New York: Parker Publishing Company, 1979.

Airola, Paavo, *Are You Confused?* Phoenix, Arizona, Health Plus Publishers, 1985.

Archives of Internal Medicine, 1998; 158:466-72.

Ban Breathnach, Sarah. *Simple Abundance.* New York, New York, Warner Books, Time Warner, 1998.

Barnard, Neal, M.D., *The Negative Calorie Effect.* McKinney, Texas, The Magni Group, 1996.

Blanchard, Kenneth, and Johnson, Spencer. *The One Minute Manager.* New York, New York, Berkley Books, 1984.

Borushek, Allan, *The Doctor's Calorie, Fat & Carbohydrate Counter.* Costa Mesa, California, Family Health Publications, 1999.

Century 21 Real Estate. *Twenty-One Ways to Tell a Winner.*

Cole-Whittaker, Terry, *21 Days to Personal Riches and Generating Wealth,* Palm Springs, California, Adventures in Enlightenment, 2000.

Cole-Whittaker, Terry, *What You Think of Me is None of My Business,* Palm Springs, California, Adventures in Enlightenment.

Covey, Stephen R. *The 7 Habits of Highly Effective People.* New York, New York, A Fireside Book, Simon & Schuster, 1990.

Diamond, Harvey & Marilyn. *Fit for Life.* New York, New York: Warner Books, 1987.

Dyer, Wayne, *Your Erroneous Zones,* New York, New York, Avon Books, Hearst Corporation, 1996.

FC&A staff, *Eat and Heal.* Peachtree City, Georgia: FC&A Medical Publishing, 2001.

Ferguson, Sarah, The Duchess of York, *Reinventing Yourself With the Duchess of York.* New York, New York, Simon and Schuster, 2001.
Hansen, Mark Victor, and Canfield, Jack, *Chicken Soup for the Unsinkable Soul.* Dearfield Beach, Florida, Health Communications, 1999.

Hansen, Mark Victor, *How to Build Your Speaking and Writing Empire.* Newport Beach, California, M.V. Hansen & Associates, 1996.

Harmony *Prosperity Laws* Cards.www.prosperitycards.com

Howard, Karen, *When Reason Fails...Understanding Bereavement by Suicide.* Creative Marketing, Springfield, Illinois, 1982.

International Journal of Obesity and Related Metabolic Disorders, 1998; 22:39-47
Journal of American Medical Association, 1997; 278:1407-11.

Judd, H.S.; Terrill, James M.; and Langenwalter, Evelyn, *California Weight Loss Program.* Palo Alto, California, HSJ Publishers, 1974.

Kamen, Betty. *Hormone Replacement Therapy Yes or No?* Novato, California, Nutrition Encounter, 1993.

Livingston, Carole, *I'll Never Be Fat Again.* Secaucus, New Jersey, Lyle Stuart Inc., 1980.

McGinnis JM, Foege WH, *Actual Causes of Death in the United States, Journal of the American Medical Association, 1993: 270: 2207-12.*

Mackay, Harvey, *Swim With the Sharks,* New York, New York, William Morrow and Company, 1998.
McGraw, Dr. Phil, *Life Strategies,* New York, New York, Hyperion, 1999.

Mellin, Laurel, *The Solution,* New York, New York, Harper Collins Publishers, 1997.

New England Journal of Medicine, 1999; 341:1097-105.

Parry, Bob, Director Chaplaincy Services. *Life Goes On.* Hoag Memorial Hospital, Newport Beach, California.

Ramirez, Judy, Bereavement Counselor, St. Simon and Jude Catholic Church, Huntington Beach, California.

Robbins, Tony, *Personal Power!* Irwindale, California, Guthy-Renker Corporation, 1989.

Robbins, Tony, *Awaken the Giant Within,* New York, New York, Fireside, Simon and Schuster, 1991.

Ruiz, Don Miguel, *The Four Agreements*, San Rafael, California, Amber-Allen Publishing, 2000.

Satcher, Dr. David; *Surgeon General's Report on Overweight and Obesity,* December 13, 2001.

St. Bonaventure Bereavement Ministry. Huntington Beach, California.

VanTine, Julia; Doherty, Bridget, and Editors of Prevention Health Books for Women, *Growing Younger.* Rodale and St. Martin's Press, 1999.

Williamson, Marianne, *A Return to Love, poem: Our Deepest Fear. 1996*

Winfrey, Oprah, *The Uncommon Wisdom of Oprah Winfrey,* Secaucus, New Jersey, Citadel Press Book, Carol Publishing Group, 1996.

Yeager, Selene and the Editors of Prevention Health Books, *New Foods for Healing.* New York, New York: Bantam Books with Rodale Press, 1999.

INDEX

For information about inviting
Jean Krueger to speak to an
Organization, conference, church,
Retreat or event
Please contact:

WHY THE WEIGHT? Dare to Be Great!
Jean Krueger
211 18 Street
Huntington Beach, California 92648
Phone: (714)-536-0408
Fax: (714)-536-0408
Email: skinnyjean@mindspring.com
www.allcalifspeakers.com

QUICK ORDER FORM
(Permission granted for duplication of this page.)

Email orders: skinnyjean@mindspring.com
www.allcalifspeakers.com
Fax orders: 714-536-0408
Telephone orders: call 714-536-0408
Postal orders: *WHY THE WEIGHT? Dare to Be Great!*
Jean Krueger
211 18 Street, Huntington Beach, California 92648.
Telephone: 714-536-0408

Please send me the following books, reports or tapes. I understand that I may return any of them for a full refund—for any reason, no questions asked.*

____**$15.95** ***WHY THE WEIGHT? Dare to Be Great! (Book)***
____**$5.00** "The Magic In You" (report)
____**$5.00** "The New You: Body, Mind and Spirit" (report)
____**$5.00** "The Final Insult" (report)
____**$5.00** "Four Agreements Will Change Your World" (report)
____**$5.00** "How to Eat More—Yet Weigh Less!" (report)
____**$6.00** "Foods to Eat More—Yet Weigh Less!" (report)
____**$5.00** "The Seven Keys To a **SLIMMER** New You!" (report)
____**$5.00** "I Can Do It!" (report)
____**$5.00** "Skinny Jean's" Secrets (report)
____**$5.00** "Skinny Jean's" Strategies (report)
(The reports listed above are reprints of individual chapters from the book:
WHY THE WEIGHT? Dare To Be Great!)
____**$5.00** "I Can Do It!" Affirmations (audio tape)
____**$15.95** ***WHY THE WEIGHT? Dare to Be Great!*** (audio tapes)
____**$6.00** ***ENDORSEMENTS: Jump Your Book Out of the Box!*** (report)
Please send more FREE information on Jean's:
☐Other Books ☐Speaking/Seminars ☐Mailing lists ☐Consulting

Name: _____
Address_____
City_____State_____Zip_____
Telephone_____
email address_____

_____**Sales tax: Please add 7.75 % % for products shipped to California addresses.**
_____**Shipping in U.S.: $3.50 for first book or product, and $2.00 for each additional product.**
_____**Shipping International: send actual cost.**
_____**Total**

Payment: ___check ___**credit card:**
__**Visa** ___**MasterCard** ___**AMEX** ___**Discover**
Card number_____ **Expiration Date**____/____
Name on Card_____

*If item is returned, buyer must pay return postage.